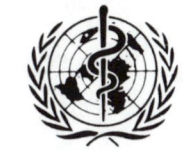

World Health Organization
  Global Network of WHO Collaborating Centres
  for Nursing/Midwifery Development

Women's Health and Development
A Global Challenge

Beverly J. McElmurry, EdD, FAAN
Kathleen F. Norr, PhD
Randy Spreen Parker, MSN, C

The University of Illinois at Chicago
College of Nursing
Chicago, Illinois

JONES AND BARTLETT PUBLISHERS
BOSTON   LONDON

Editorial, Sales, and Customer Service Offices

Jones and Bartlett Publishers
One Exeter Plaza
Boston, MA 02116

Jones and Bartlett Publishers International
PO Box 1498
London W6 7RS
England

Library of Congress Cataloging-in-Publication Data

— Data not available at time of printing

ISBN 0-086720-799-X

Acquisitions Editor: Jan Wall
Production Director: Paula Carroll
Electronic Production and Prepress: David Child
Production Editor: Anne Noonan
Cover Design: Hannus Design Associates

Cover illustration: "Drum Beat of the Earth," by Maxine Noel-Ioyan Mani.

Printed in the United States of America
97 96 95 94 93   10 9 8 7 6 5 4 3 2 1

Contents

Western Pacific

Conclusion

Preface

The theme of the Technical Discussions of the Forty-fifth Session of the World Health Assembly was Women, Health and Development. Just prior to the World Health Assembly, the Global Network of WHO Nursing Collaborating Centres met in Ferney-Voltaire, France, for its fifth Annual Network Meeting. Given the importance of developing a global perspective on women's health and development, many of the Centres agreed to develop a paper which represented either the country in which the Centre was located or a special perspective on women's health that reflected the work of the Centre. This book is a compilation of most of these reports. Although many countries are not represented here, it is our hope that in the future authors from other centres will make additional contributions to our efforts to describe women's health status. Some of the problems our authors faced were civil war, time constraints, limited resources, and availability and access to information. Moreover, some of the issues we asked our authors to write about are sensitive topics within their culture. We want to acknowledge the courage and risk some authors took to present candid information regarding women's health status within their countries.

We initially received no information from network members in Africa, so we pursued the development of chapters relevant to African countries with doctoral students associated with The University of Illinois at Chicago Nursing Collaborating Centre. They are nurses from the country they discussed or nurses with extensive experience in that country.

We are grateful for the contributions and patience of our authors as the global nursing network launched what we hope is the first of many contributions to advancing the health of women. Our editor at Jones and Bartlett, Jan Wall, made all things possible as she paved the way for our efforts. The cover by Mani was a serendipitous event in that once we saw this work of art, we knew it captured a global sense of women. The tables for some chapters were a challenge that Chang Park met with graciousness and a great deal of contributed time. David Child good naturedly took on the final formatting for the typed copy. Our sincere appreciation to all those who assisted us in this initial effort.

The preparation of this document taught us just how difficult it was to address the original outline we suggested for the description of women's health and development. Yet, nurses have an unique opportunity to advance the global health of women. There is probably no other health professional with such close, ongoing service relationships with women in all parts of the world. Combining their relationships with the advancement of primary health care education, practice, and research through nursing leadership holds the promise of giving women a voice. The editors share the common belief that listening and responding to the health concerns of women will result in better health for all people.

Beverly J. McElmurry and Kathleen F. Norr
Chicago, Illinois

Introduction

Office of Secretariat
Global Network of WHO Collaborating Centres

M. J. Kim and Virginia L. Ohlson

THE GLOBAL NETWORK OF WHO COLLABORATING CENTRES FOR NURSING DEVELOPMENT: A HISTORICAL PERSPECTIVE

WHO Collaborating Centres

With the growth of concern for women's health over the last two decades, we have developed many strategies to assist us in making our voices heard. An important tool in increasing our sensitivity to particular issues is the use of existing networks to share information and ideas. To this end the global network of nursing collaborating centres was judged an important vehicle for increasing our sensitivity to important and culturally specific issues in women's health.

By definition a WHO Collaborating Centre is an institution designated by the World Health Organization to form part of an international collaborative network carrying out activities in support of the organization's program at all levels. As implied in this definition, the purpose of any institution in its role as a WHO Collaborating Centre is to work collaboratively with the World Health Organization in support of its programs—locally, nationally, and internationally.

There are over 700 WHO Collaborating Centres located in many areas of the world and representing many, if not all, of the major health disciplines. Each Collaborating Centre negotiates with the World Health Organization in the setting of its goals and objectives as a Collaborating Centre. These goals and objectives, in the World Health Organization's terminology, are referred to as its "Terms of Reference." Objectives, or Terms of Reference, of the various Centres may differ significantly in accord with the nature or type of the institution and the particular expertise the Centre brings to the World Health Organization in carrying out its projected program. In all instances, however, designation as a WHO Collaborating Centre is given only when the institution has demonstrated that it has the scientific and technical leadership potential to work collaboratively with the World Health Organization (WHO) in carrying out the Organization's programs.

Designation as a Collaborating Centre

An institution interested in becoming a Collaborating Centre negotiates this prospect with staff of its Regional WHO Office or the WHO Headquarters in Geneva, Switzerland, and submits a proposal outlining the "plan of work" that it proposes to carry out in its role as a Collaborating Centre. In some instances the initial negotiation to become a Centre may be initiated not by the institution but by staff of WHO Regional or Headquarters Offices. Eventual designation in either instance requires three levels of approval: 1) the WHO Office of the Region in which the institution is located; 2) the prime governmental agency or office invested with international affairs in the country of the applicant; and 3) the Director General of the WHO Headquarters Office in Geneva, Switzerland.

Although the designation of institutions and agencies as WHO Collaborating Centres is not a new activity, it is only recently that this recognition has been given to nursing institutions. The earliest nursing Collaborating Centres to be so identified were in Europe, when in the early 1980s the European Regional Office of the WHO (EURO) designated seven nursing institutions or agencies of Europe to serve as regional advisory/teaching-learning Centres to stimulate within Europe the progress of nursing research and, specifically, nursing practice.

The Development of the Global Network
of Who Collaborating Centres for Nursing

The establishment of the Network dates back to March of 1987, to an interregional workshop convened by the WHO Headquarters to discuss the potential of establishing a global network of nursing institutions and organizations that would work together for nursing's development in support of the goal of "Health for All" through Primary Health Care. The workshop was envisioned and planned by Dr. Amelia Maglacas, who was then the Chief Scientist for Nursing at WHO Headquarters and hosted by the Nursing Colleges Division of the Thailand Ministry of Health. Twenty-three nursing leaders representing 20 different institutions, agencies, and organizations were present at this workshop, a number of which are now represented in the membership of the Network. At the time of the workshop only five nursing institutions had been designated as WHO Collaborating Centres, four of the original regional Centres of Europe (Finland, Denmark, France, and Yugoslavia) and one new global Centre in the USA (Illinois). It was a productive 3-day meeting culminating "in the unanimous agreement to establish a global network of WHO Collaborating Centres for Nursing Development as an integral part of national and international strategies for achieving 'Health for All' by the Year 2000 through Primary Health Care." (1)   It was unanimously agreed at that time that the Secretariat of the Network would be located at The University of Illinois at Chicago, College of Nursing, USA and remain there initially for a 5-year period with the Dean of the College (the Collaborating Centre) functioning as the Secretary General.

Many important, complex issues were raised by the participants relating to the goals and objectives of the proposed network—its functions, organizational structure, potential resources, and possibilities for funding. An action plan was formulated and accepted. An Ad Hoc Executive Committee, appointed by the WHO, was charged with finalizing the plan and using it to draft a set of rules that would express the goals, objectives, and functions of the Network and give direction to its organization, structure, and governance. Records of the Bangkok meeting and the work of the Ad Hoc Executive Committee are in the files of the Secretariat—interesting, informative documents which describe the process that laid down the foundations for the Network and the issues related to its establishment. Some of these issues still remain, as the Network has tried to move aggressively with an action-oriented plan of work in spite of continuing funding problems to support its proposed, ever-expanding agenda.

The First General Meeting of the Network, beginning with a festive Inaugural Ceremony, was held in Maribor, Slovenia, April 20-23, 1988, hosted by the Yugoslavian Government. Forty-eight persons were in attendance, representing 22 countries and all 6 WHO Regions of the world. Since the time of the Bangkok Workshop, six new Collaborating Centres for Nursing Development in Primary Health Care had been designated by the WHO—in Australia, India, Korea, Thailand, and the USA (Pennsylvania and Texas). Prime matters of business at this meeting dealt with the purpose of the Network, its goals and objectives, plan of work, and the rules for the operation of the Network. A draft of the Constitution and By-laws was prepared and accepted in principle for use as a guiding document until it might be further considered and accepted at the next General Meeting of the Network.

By the time of the Second General Meeting of the Network, held in Copenhagen, Denmark, August 2 and 3, 1989, significant personnel changes had occurred in the top nursing leadership position at the WHO Headquarters in Geneva, at the Collaborating Centre in Denmark that was hosting the meeting, and at the University of Illinois at Chicago, College of Nursing, the Secretariat for the Network. Dr. Miriam Hirschfeld had been appointed Chief Scientist for Nursing at the WHO Headquarters following the retirement of Dr. Amelia Maglacas who had provided the idea and initial leadership for the establishment of the Network. Dr. Mi Ja Kim, newly appointed Dean of the College of Nursing, University of Illinois at Chicago, had assumed directorship of the Secretariat as Secretary General of the Network. Ms. Randi Mortensen, newly appointed Director of the Denmark Collaborating Centre, chaired the meeting. Thirty-eight persons representing 21 countries were present. Since the First General Meeting of the Network, two University Schools of Nursing had been newly designated as WHO Collaborating Centres—in Brazil and the Philippines. The Global Network was growing. By the time of this meeting, 13 nursing institutions and agencies had been designated as WHO Collaborating Centres for Nursing Development in Primary Health Care—in all WHO areas of the world except the African and Eastern Mediterranean Regions. It was at this General Meeting that the Constitution and Bylaws, as debated and drafted at the Bangkok Workshop and at the meeting in Slovenia were finalized and accepted, setting down the guiding rules for the Network, and most importantly, its statement of purpose, goals, and objectives.

THE PURPOSE, GOALS, AND OBJECTIVES OF THE NETWORK

Purpose

There shall be a Global Network of WHO Collaborating Centres for Nursing, and its central purpose is to strengthen and promote nursing leadership towards the realization of the social goal of 'Health for All through Primary Health Care'. This shall be achieved through a process of collaborating, coordination, and mobilization of resources in the areas of nursing education, research and practice. (Constitution of the Network)

Goal

The Network has as its primary *goal* the strengthening of membership institutions in their efforts to improve nursing development including education, practice, research and leadership—to achieve the goal of Health for All through Primary Health Care. (Bylaws of the Network)

Objectives

1) Strengthen the education, service and research programs of the Network's members aimed at the goal of Health for All.
2) Develop appropriate technologies (approaches, tools and methodologies) for nursing development that emphasize primary health care.
3) Promote the expanded role of nursing in the implementation of Health for All strategies in health services delivery and educational programs.
4) Exchange information among Collaborating Centres to introduce innovations in health manpower development.
5) Collaborate with relevant governmental and nongovernmental organizations in the achievement of the goals and objectives of the Network.
6) Liaise with relevant groups to strengthen Network activities. (Bylaws of the Network) (2)

Following the two organizational meetings in Slovenia and Denmark, three annual meetings were held—in Galveston, Texas, USA in 1990, in Geneva, Switzerland in 1991, and in Ferney-Voltaire, France in 1992. Each year newly designated WHO Nursing Collaborating Centres were added to the Network membership. At the time of this writing, 22 nursing institutions and agencies had been designated as Members of the Global Network of WHO Collaborating Centres for Nursing Development in Primary Health Care (see Box below.)

Membership in the Network also includes the International Council of Nurses (ICN), the Chief Scientist for Nursing of the WHO Headquarters and the six Regional Nurse Officers Offices of WHO, two Honorary Members and a few Associate Members in process of designation as WHO Collaborating Centres for Nursing Development.

The global Network for Nursing Development in Primary Health Care has grown rapidly. It is now already 6 years old. Its goals are quite clear and its potential for leadership increasingly is being recognized. There has been a lot of "give and take" between members, and a good amount of exchange and sharing of resources and personnel. Dissemination of the work of our collaborative Network has only just begun but remains before us as a continuing challenge. This book on the health status of women in selected countries represents efforts of the network members to prepare papers consistent with the theme of the 1992 WHO technical sessions. These sessions, held prior to the annual meeting of the WHO Assembly, provide an opportunity for representatives of member countries to focus on shared health concerns. Network members agree with the WHO statement, "that women's health status has an important impact in the health of their children, the family, the community and the environment." (3)

REFERENCES

1. *Report of the Secretariat to the 1992 General Meeting of the Global Network of WHO Collaborating Centres for Nursing Development in PHC.* This and other reports are available in the files of the Secretariat, College of Nursing, University of Illinois at Chicago.
2. *Constitution and Bylaws of the Global Network for Nursing Development in Primary Health Care.* Chicago: In the files of the Secretariat, College of Nursing, University of Illinois at Chicago, (Unpublished document), 1990.
3. WHO. (1992). *Women's health: Across age and frontier.* World Health Organization.

MEMBERS OF THE GLOBAL NETWORK
OF WHO COLLABORATING CENTRES
FOR NURSING DEVELOPMENT
IN PRIMARY HEALTH CARE
AS OF MARCH 1993

Africa

Universite de Kinshasa
    Institute Superieur des Techniques Medicales
    Collaborating Centre for the Development of Nursing Services
    Kinshasa, Zaire
University of Botswana
    Department of Nursing Education
    Collaborating Centre for Nursing Development Towards HFA/PHC
    Gaborone, Botswana

Americas

The Colombian Association of Schools and Colleges of Nursing
    Collaborating Centre for Nursing Development in Primary Health Care
    Santafe de Bogota D.E., Colombia
George Mason University
    School of Nursing
    Collaborating Centre for Nursing Administration, Health Policy and Health
        Care Ethics
    Fairfax, Virginia, USA
McMaster University
    School of Nursing
    Collaborating Centre for Nursing
    Hamilton, Ontario, Canada
University of California at San Francisco
    School of Nursing
    Collaborating Centre for Research and Clinical Training in Nursing
    San Francisco, California, USA
The University of Illinois at Chicago
    College of Nursing
    Collaborating Centre for International Nursing Development in Primary Health
        Care
    Chicago, Illinois, USA
University of Pennsylvania
    School of Nursing
    Collaborating Centre for International Nursing Development in Research,
        Leadership and Education
    Philadelphia, Pennsylvania, USA

University of São Paulo at Ribeirão Preto
  College of Nursing
  Collaborating Centre for Development of Nursing Research Campus de
    Ribeirão Preto
  Ribeirão Preto, SP, Brazil
University of Texas Medical Branch
  School of Nursing
  Collaborating Centre for Nursing Development
  Galveston, Texas, USA

Eastern Mediterranean

Nursing Division - College of Health Sciences
  Ministry of Health - State of Bahrain
  Collaborating Centre for Nursing Development
  Manama, Bahrain

Europe

The Danish Institute for Health and Nursing Research
  Collaborating Centre for Nursing Research and Education
  Copenhagen, Denmark
Health Centre
  Collaborating Centre for Primary Health Care Nursing
  Maribor, Slovenia
Hospices Civils de Lyon
  Collaborating Centre in Nursing
  Lyon, France
Nursing and International Health Unit
  Collaborating Centre for Primary Health Care and Nursing
  Alma Ata, Kazakhstan
The Supporting Association of the
  Nursing Research Institute in Finland
  Collaborating Centre for Nursing
  Helsinki, Finland
University of Manchester
  Queen's Nursing Institute
  Collaborating Centre for Reference, Education and Research in Primary
    Health Care Nursing
  Manchester, United Kingdom

South-East Asia

Ministry of Public Health
    Nursing College Division
    Collaborating Centre for Nursing Development Toward HFA/PHC
    Bangkok, Thailand
Rajkumari Amrit Kaur College of Nursing
    Collaborating Centre for Nursing Development
    New Delhi, India

Western Pacific

St. Luke's College of Nursing
    Collaborating Centre for Nursing Development in Primary Health Care
    Tokyo, Japan
University of the Philippines
    College of Nursing
    Collaborating Centre for Nursing Development in Primary Health Care
    Manila, Philippines
The University of Sydney
    Cumberland College of Health Sciences
    Collaborating Centre for Nursing Development in PHC
    Lidcombe, N.S.W., Australia
Yonsei University
    College of Nursing
    Collaborating Centre for Nursing Development
    Seoul, Korea

Overview

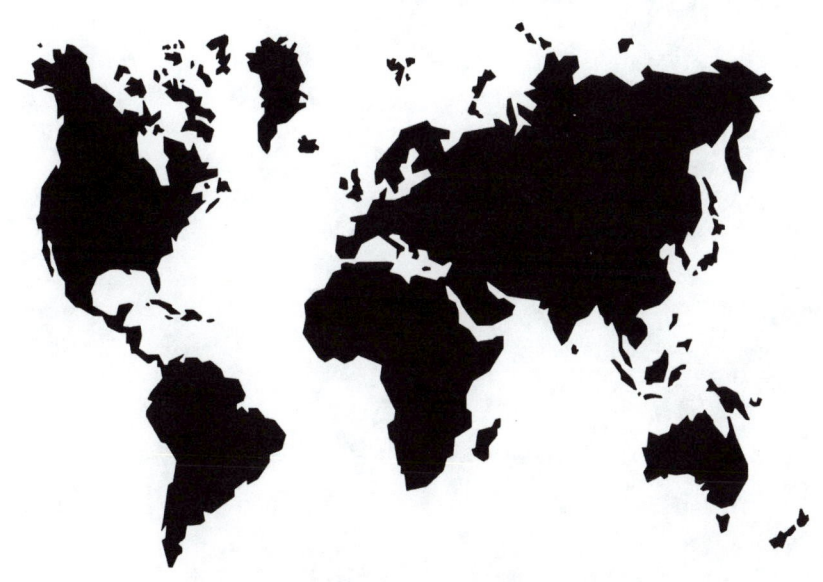

Women's
Health Status
Across the Globe

Women's Health Status Across the Globe

Beverly J. McElmurry, Kathleen F. Norr, Randy Spreen Parker

Women's health and development is a phrase used throughout this book to depict the complex interrelationship between the health of women and their social, political, cultural, and economic situation. The meaning of women's health and development has changed over time with an initial emphasis on equity, human rights, and welfare issues, such as women in poverty, to a broader meaning that focused on the economic growth and contribution of women. More recently, the notion of women's health and development has expanded to include an emphasis on empowerment and global development goals and mechanisms that enable women to gain greater control over their lives (Women in Development, 1992). This more inclusive and holistic definition best captures our emerging conception of women's health and development. This approach reflects a shift away from a view of women as victims and passive objects toward an understanding of women as independent actors capable of constructing knowledge and affecting change grounded in their lived experiences. Thus, the health status of women affects not only the health of their children and other family members but also their contribution to the welfare of their communities and societies.

Women's health is an integral part of the overall development of a nation. The current health status of women is strongly influenced by the level of development. At the same time, improving women's health is an important component of overall development. Improving women's health contributes to development both directly, through the economic and social contributions of the women themselves, and indirectly, through their contribution to the health and welfare of their families. In the abstract, this statement has become a familiar platitude. Yet, each of the countries described in this volume provides clear evidence of the link between women's health and development in many different countries and regions.

The poorer the country is overall, the fewer resources there are to be devoted to women's health. Although some issues, such as violence and reproductive health, affect all women, the characteristic health problems of women differ in developing and industrialized nations. The most pressing women's health needs in developing countries are those associated with a relatively young population, a moderate to high birth rate and a declining death rate, safe motherhood, and infectious/contagious diseases. In more industrialized countries, a low birth and death rate and an aging population mean that women face more problems related to chronic and degenerative conditions.

While a country's overall level of development clearly affects women's health, the authors' descriptions of women's health around the world identify two other important factors: the cultural position and current political system as they relate to women. Gender discrimination is a worldwide phenomenon, but specific gender discrimination patterns very widely. For example, in some countries women are restricted in their freedom of movement, while in others women play important public roles as traders or marketers. The current and past political system's level of commitment to health and/or equality also affects the degree of resources committed to women's health. The opportunity to participate in political activities gives women a chance to organize their own interests. Political violence and oppression usually have profound negative impacts on women's health. Other factors contributing to women's health problems include early childbearing, lack of education, lack of economic opportunity, and lower wages for the same work.

COMPARISON BY REGION

To assist authors in describing the status of women's health for their chapters, McElmurry and Norr developed a comprehernsive outline to examine women's health and development. The Guide to Women's Health Status (Box 1-1) was shared with the Global Nursing Network members with the request that they use the Guide to portray women in their country. Also, the Appendix contains the Congress Statement of the delegates to the Fifth International Congress on Women Health Issues, which they adopted August 28, 1992, in Copenhagen, Denmark. This document is included because its statement of international priorities underscores the concerns of Network members.

A comparison of women's health in the six World Health Organization regions (Africa, the Americas, Eastern Mediterranean, Europe, South-East Asia, Western Pacific) highlights both the common concerns women face throughout the world and the unique challenges of specific countries. The countries comprising the WHO regions, along with the address of the regional office, are found in Box 1-2 at the end of this chapter.

Africa is the world's poorest region today, lacking both money and trained personnel. Many countries cannot meet even the most basic health needs of their population. Sub-Saharan Africa has a very complex set of cultural traditions stemming from the customs of many different ethnic divisions and tribes, along with more recent influences of Islam and Christianity as well as colonial domination by European powers. Parts of the continent have a long tradition of women's active participation in the economy. Health needs for women center around reproduction and motherhood. Many women lack access to safer sex, family planning, and maternal child health services. High maternal and infant mortality, AIDS and other untreated sexually transmitted diseases, traditional female genital mutilations, unwanted pregnancies, and preventable problems of pregnancy are all major health concerns. The serious impact of political violence on women is highlighted in the chapter on Liberia.

Europe is a region having two distinct parts: Western Europe with its highly industrialized wealthy and democratic states and Eastern Europe and the former USSR. In Western Europe the woman's movement has a long history of struggle for equality, and women today enjoy many benefits of that struggle. Most nations have state-supported and well financed health care systems. The collapse of the former Soviet Union (USSR) and the regimes it supported has plunged many Eastern European societies into political and economic turmoil. The state-financed health care system, already unresponsive to many women's health issues, has also been seriously damaged in many countries. Renewed ethnic violence is a serious threat to the health of women in some parts of the region. Major health problems for women throughout Europe are those associated with the "double burden" of the working woman, the problems of aging and the needs of immigrant and refugee women. Eastern European women face additional concerns related to violence, reproductive health, and environmental health threats.

The Americas are a region of great diversity. The United States and Canada have many characteristics in common with Western Europe and similar health problems. However, two factors contribute to special health concerns for women in the United States. Lack of a national health or insurance plan leaves many women unable to afford even the most basic health care. Persistent societal discrimination against minority groups means that minority women face a double burden that adversely affects their health and welfare. Latin America contains a wide diversity of countries, seriously under-represented by the chapters here. Latin America as a whole shares a long tradition of Catholicism and machismo, or male domination and restriction of the woman's role to the family. Health issues especially relevant to women in Latin America include reproductive issues, especially the right to family planning, safer sex to prevent AIDS and STDs, safe motherhood, and domestic violence.

The Eastern Mediterranean is a complex region that includes the oil producing Islamic states commonly identified with the Middle East, as well as many volatile countries in the north and coastal areas of Africa. The differences between countries in this region cannot be fully represented by one chapter. However, the women of the region face enormous challenges to their health due to wars, economic hardships, and the social status of women. Many women in the Mideast have inadequate health care. There is a profound interplay between religious beliefs and health practices.

South-East Asia is a region where explosive economic growth has taken place over the last three decades. Women there have health needs that represent a mix of the health needs of developing and industrial countries. In some countries of the region, growing economic capacity has been accompanied by improvements in the health status of women, while in other countries health has not been an area of investment. Women in those countries continue to face some of the health problems of developing countries, and problems of more industrialized countries are also beginning.

The Western Pacific has had dramatic economic growth since World War II, and many of its countries are heavily industrialized. In both Korea and Japan, the health, economic, and social problems of an aging population are growing, and because women live longer than men, these issues are especially relevant to women. Australia has had these problems for a longer period of time. Women in industrialized societies also now face the health burden of the "double duty" syndrome that requires women to work outside the home and also to continue to fulfill all their traditional family responsibilities. Those countries in this region which are not represented in this document, such as China and Viet Nam, are areas where women's health issues reflect those of less developed countries.

SUMMARY

Overall, when the global health needs of women are considered, there are four areas of pressing health needs for women throughout the world:
- Safe motherhood,
- Reduction of violence against women,
- Control over one's body including prevention and management of AIDS, and
- Midlife and aging health concerns

Safe motherhood is perhaps the clearest priority in women's health. It is well established that relatively low cost and simple measures can dramatically improve survival rates and reduce morbidities for mothers and their infants. Sadly, many countries throughout the world do not yet provide these basic services. Even in highly developed countries there are often subgroups of women who receive less than adequate care, such as minority group members in the United States and immigrant women in Europe. Related to safe motherhood is the growing need women have throughout the world to find new ways of combining motherhood and work. Lack of adequate childcare or family leave opportunities threaten the physical and psychological welfare of mothers, children, and families. These problems affect women at many different economic levels and in many different countries and create high stress levels.

Violence affects women's health everywhere in the world today. No society is free of domestic violence, and many otherwise progressive societies have failed to address this problem adequately. There is still tolerance of domestic violence that in many societies would be considered a major crime if committed outside a marriage relationship. Women also suffer rape and other violent crime in far too many countries. Rape is especially problematic in many of the world's large cities. The political violence of war, civil disturbances, and communal riots, and political repression also claim many women and children as their victims. In an increasingly unstable world, regions once thought stable are now rocked with violence.

Control over one's body is a broad area encompassing many related concerns. Issues related to sexuality have been especially resistant to change because different societies have a wide variety of beliefs and practices that affect women's sexual behaviors. To achieve health, women need to have their sexuality respected and need the right to exercise control over their bodies. Female genital mutilation is one example of a serious threat to women's health. Equally urgent today is the right of every woman to have safer sex to protect herself from AIDS, other STDs and unintended childbearing. Unsafe abortion is also a serious threat to women's health that needs to be considered.

Health needs related to midlife and aging are becoming increasingly important as women's life spans increase. Specific health concerns for women include understanding and normalizing the menopause experience, prevention and early treatment of the most prevalent women's cancers, especially breast and cervical cancer, and more attention to the physical, psychological, social, and economic aspects of aging. As death rates decline, women in nearly all countries live longer than men, and the problems of aging become especially relevant for women.

Women have made great progress in demanding and obtaining better health. Women also have many unfinished tasks and continuing health problems. In many cases, improving women's health requires social and economic changes. Clear examples include reduction of early childbearing; increased education and economic opportunities; overcoming traditional beliefs and values that have negative consequences for women's health, such as genital mutilation and restriction of knowledge about safer sex; and increased political representation of women's interests. Improving women's health is compatible with a primary health care approach. Alternatively, primary health care's emphasis on equality, access, and participation and its prevention focus, will help to ensure that women receive their fair share of health care services.

REFERENCES

Women in Development, (1992). *Women 2000, 1*, p. 4.

Box 1-1. Guide to Women's Health Status

Synopsis of Country

Area, population, form of government, major health concerns.

Demographics

Language, races, or other ethnic divisions, literacy rates by gender and age, birth rates, death rates, infant mortality rates and life expectancy overall and for men and women; sex ratio at birth and at later ages.

Health Care System/Financing

Type of system (public-private-mixed); if a traditional care system exists and how widespread, whether integrated into "Western" system, any descriptions of traditional practices, especially as they affect women; if PHC model used and if so, how; number of different kinds of health workers and number per capita, how distributed geographically (e.g., urban/rural, regional differences); level of expenditure, expenditure per capita, and any available information on spending by specific problems of regions. Is there any pattern of lower expenditure on problems that are more often suffered by women?

Health Service Utilization

Number of women receiving prenatal care, where babies are born, and any other basic coverage statistics, if possible by gender, rural-urban and region where relevant; any available data on number of referrals from rural to higher level facilities, clinic visits per capita, etc. In essence, are access and acceptability of services an influence on the women's use of health services?

Educational Achievement for Women

Whatever is available about male/female ratios at different levels of school; number of female graduates in advanced degrees and ratio to men.

Economics

Per capita income; degree of inequality of wealth; percent female headed households and income differential; percent of women and children in poverty in comparison to men; labor force participation rates for women compared to men; types of occupations where women are located, with special focus on agricultural sector, family unpaid labor; property ownership by women; any legal or customary restrictions on women's economic participation; inheritance laws; welfare, pension, retirement schemes and degree of participation by women in them.

Family Structure

Marriage laws; percent married; age at marriage; customary brideprice or dowry, arranged marriage; birth rates, average intervals between births, breastfeeding prevalence and duration; divorce law, divorce rates, division of property and rights for children of divorce; what happens to widows— restrictions, rights, etc.

Sexuality

Female circumcision, mutilation; customary degree of restriction of movement of women and any differences by region, social class, or age; contraceptive laws and practices; abortion laws and practices, number of deaths from septic abortion; pornography; extent of commercial sex and criminalization of women but not men, forced prostitution, etc.

Violence Against Women

Spouse abuse, rape, incest, women in prison.

Women's Strengths

Women's political and social organizations, etc.

Political Participation of Women

If the population votes for officials, percent of males, females who vote; number and proportion of women in elected and appointed government offices; participation of women in national and regional political parties and other organizations; any women's political organizations and activities such as conferences, protests, etc. Whether women are in the military; if subject to draft; what roles they play in military.

Other Aspects of Interest to Women's Health

Box 1-2. WHO Regions and Regional Offices as of March 1993

Africa
WHO/Regional Office for Africa
P.O.B. 6, Brazzaville, Congo
Algeria, Angola, Benin, Botswana, Burkina Faso, Burundi, Cameroon, Cape Verde, Central African Republic, Chad, Comoros, Congo, Côte D'Ivoire, Equatorial Guinea, Ethiopia, Gabon, Gambin, Ghana, Guinea, Guinea-Bissau, Kenya, Lesotho, Liberia, Madagascar, Malawi, Mali, Mauritania, Mauritius, Mozambique, Namibia, Niger, Nigeria, Rwanda, Sao Tome and Principe, Senegal, Seychelles, Sierra Leone, South Africa, Swaziland, Togo, Uganda, United Republic of Tanzania, Zaire, Zambia, Zimbabwe.

Americas
WHO/Regional Office for the Americas/Pan American Sanitary Bureau (PAHO)
525 23rd Street, N.W.
Washington, D.C. 20037, USA
Antigua and Barbuda, Argentina, Bahamas, Barbados, Belize, Bolivia, Brazil, Canada, Chile, Colombia, Costa Rica, Cuba, Dominica, Dominican Republic, Ecuador, El Salvador, Grenada, Guatemala, Guyana, Haiti, Honduras, Jamaica, Mexico, Nicaragua, Panama, Paraguay, Peru, Saint Kitts and Nevis, Saint Lucia, Saint Vincent and the Grenadines, Suriname, Trinidad and Tobago, United States of America, Uruguay, Venezuela.

Eastern Mediterranean
WHO/Regional Office for the Eastern Mediterranean
P.O. Box 1517
Alexandria - 21511, Egypt
Afghanistan, Bahrain, Cyprus, Djibouti, Egypt, Iran (Islamic Republic of), Iraq, Jordan, Kuwait, Lebanon, Libyan Arab Jamahiriya, Morocco, Oman, Pakistan, Qatar, Saudi Arabia, Somalia, Sudan, Syrian Arab Republic, Tunisia, United Arab Emirates, Yemen.

Europe
WHO/Regional Office for Europe
8, Scherfigsvej
2100 Copenhagen 0, Denmark
Albania, Armenia, Austria, Azerbaijan, Belarus, Belgium, Bosnia and Herzegovina, Bulgaria, Croatia, Czech Repulic, Denmark, Finland, France, Georgia, Germany, Greece, Hungary, Iceland, Ireland, Israel, Italy, Kazakhstan, Kyrgyzstan, Latvia, Lithuania, Luxembourg, Malta, Monaco, Netherlands, Norway, Poland, Portugal, Republic of Moldova, Romania, Russian Federation, San Marino, Slovak Republic, Slovenia, Spain, Sweden, Switzerland, Tajikistan, Turkey, Turkmenistan, Ukraine, United Kingdom of Great Britain and Northern Ireland, Uzbekistan, Yugoslavia.

South-East Asia
WHO/Regional Office for South-East Asia
World Health House; Indraprastha Estate
Mahatma Gandhi Road
New Delhi-110002, India
Bangladesh, Bhutan, Democratic People's Republic of Korea, India, Indonesia, Maldives, Mongolia, Myanmar, Nepal, Sri Lanka, Thailand.

Western Pacific
WHO/Regional Office for the Western Pacific
P.O. Box 2932
1099 Manila, Philippines
Australia, Brunei Darussalam, Cambodia, China, Cook Islands, Fiji, Japan, Kiribati, Lao People's Democratic Republic, Malaysia, Marshall Islands, Micronesia (Federated States of), New Zealand, Papua New Guinea, Philippines, Republic of Korea, Samoa, Singapore, Solomon Islands, Tonga, Vanuatu, Viet Nam.

Africa

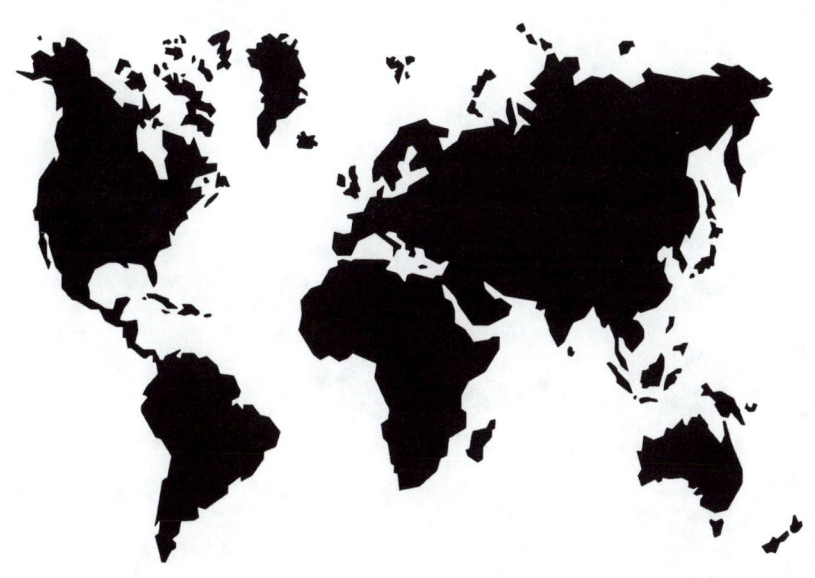

**Liberia
Nigeria
South Africa**

Women's Health Status in Liberia

Associated with The University of Illinois at Chicago WHO Collaborating Centre

Aaron G. Buseh

INTRODUCTION

"In most Countries of Africa, whole sectors of the economy, such as internal trade, agriculture, agro-business, and health care are in the hands of women" (*West Africa Magazine*, September 9-15, 1991). This chapter attempts to outline the Liberian woman and her many plights as she goes through her daily activities. A brief overview of Liberia is given in the paper which should enlighten the reader on the background of Liberia and how it came to be what it is today. The health delivery system, health care financing, health manpower training, and deployment will also be discussed. The paper emphasizes the Liberian woman, her educational status and socioeconomic status. Other issues discussed in this manuscript are the family structure, sexuality and contraceptive knowledge and use, violence against women, and women's participation in public life and leadership. Finally, this chapter describes the impact of the Liberian civil war on the health of women and children.

I have tried to create some distinction between women either by their educational status, area of residence i.e., rural or urban. Each of these groups could be stratified and looked at differently. One common error sociologists have made in analyzing Liberian society is to lump all women into one homogeneous group, perhaps seeking to demonstrate female solidarity in the face of male oppression. However, I think it is fair to say that women in Liberia do share some common characteristics.

If we begin by looking at rural traditional women in Liberia, we shall see that their economic roles are closely related to their marital options and constraints. Some sociologists who have studied African cultures argue that because of the dominant role of African women in production, they are highly independent, mobile and able to accumulate wealth and status on their own. But this is not true for all women. In fact the extent of women's dominance in the farming process with regard to decision-making needs to be questioned. Men in Liberia and many other Sub-Saharan countries in Africa dominate both traditional female farming systems as well as the modern markets and make these institutions serve their own interests. Marriage, then, could be suggested as the main vehicle for this economic subordination of women in the Liberian culture. As a matter of fact, many of the women's efforts on the farm enter the men's pocket.

Modernization in Liberia and around the world has definitely provided opportunities for women to acquire status, independence, and prestige. For example, where cash cropping is possible or wage labor opportunities are available, women can remain unmarried because cash from marketing or from wage-earning lovers can be used to hire farm labor, pay house taxes, and buy household necessities themselves. This pattern may be similar in other African countries. More than men, women seem to be able to cooperate, to stand by each other even in difficult times and to follow a common aim.

Traditionally (probably in all the Liberian ethnic groups), e.g., the Kpelle tribe, only a few women hold legal rights in themselves or in others. Ordinarily, women do not have the right to expect others to prepare their meals, heat their bath water, or clean their clothes. They also do not have rights to bridewealth or brideservice from their children's marriage. On the other hand, a man in the Kpelle culture acquires domestic support for his ambitions in the public realm simply by birthright and by marriage. A woman seeking political advancement thus begins with a double handicap. Advancement requires her to retain the benefits of her labor reproduction, but marriage and the legal system fix her to the domestic realm and the benefits of her services to man. Hence, women in Liberia must work much harder than men to derive support from the domestic sphere.

Information compiled in this manuscript has been taken from a variety of sources including the Ministry of Health and Social Welfare Annual Report, the Ministry of Planning and Economic Affairs Annual Reports, and several World Bank publications. The quality of statistical information varied greatly, a problem not unique to Liberia but common in several developing countries. Available information was often noted to be incomplete and at times conflicting. Such data limitations do not prevent my discussing the profile of women's health and development in Liberia. It is a very important topic and I am glad I had the opportunity to do it. It was also an exciting learning experience for me. It must finally be noted that most of the information used here are data from the late 1980s. The breakdown of the government in Liberia in 1990 made it impossible for relevant information to be collected in the area of health.

OVERVIEW OF LIBERIA

Liberia is one of the oldest republics on the continent of Africa and is unique because of its noncolonial background. Available information suggests that the spatial settlement of various ethnic groups found today began sometime in the 14th century. European explorers and seafarers frequented the west coast of Africa during the 15th century. The Europeans (e.g., Portuguese, French, British, and Dutch) came to Liberia in search of items for trade, including ivory, gold, and malegueta pepper.

In 1822, emancipated slaves from the United States of American began arriving in Liberia. This marked the beginning of a new era for Liberia. They brought new cultures and values acquired while in slavery. Even to the present day it has not been easy for the freed slaves known as "Americo-Liberians" to settle with the indigenous population. The Americo-Liberians constituted about 3% of the country's population but governed the country on a colonial pattern of indirect rule, thus transferring the socioeconomic and political systems of the United States to Liberia. After more than a century of settlers' oligarchy, a change took place in Liberia's political structure. On April 12, 1980, a coup d'etat ushered the first indigenous leader. This was the start of what is known as the Second Republic.

The indigenous people of Liberia comprise about 96% of the country's population and are identified into 16 major tribes. Since the military coup in 1980, there has been a series of attempts to overthrow the government. The government was accused of rampant corruption and abuse of human rights. In December 1989, rebels under the leadership of Mr. Charles Taylor invaded the modern part of the country which led to one of the worst civil wars in the history of Africa. General Samuel Doe was killed and his body mutilated. Since then, the country has not returned to normal. Various factions continue to fight for power and 40,000 lives have been lost.

Geography and Climate

Liberia is located on the west coast of Africa. It covers an area of approximately 99,068 square kilometers. It is bordered by Sierra Leone on the west, Guinea on the north, and the Ivory coast on the east. On the south is the Atlantic Ocean, with a long coastline of 550 kilometers. The climate is humid tropical, with a long rainy season lasting from April to October and a dry season from

November to March. The average annual temperature is 28°C due to climatic conditions; Liberia has a tropical rain forest vegetation.

Economy

Prior to civil war in 1990, Liberia's economy had been considerably influenced by the importation of raw materials, equipment, and a wide variety of consumer goods. The most important activity is the mining and shipment of iron ore. But due to declining economic world demand, its share of the export market has decreased considerably. Other exports include rubber, timber, diamonds, and increasingly, agricultural commodities. About 70% of the Liberian population is engaged in traditional agriculture, growing rice, cocoa, coffee, and other cash crops. Because of low yields and moderate income, this sector has little influence on the economy as a whole.

Population

According to the last Population and Housing Census conducted in 1984, the population of Liberia was estimated to be 2.463 million people. The estimated annual growth rate is 3.1%. This will yield a 46% increase in total population by the year 2000, according to Ministry Of Planning and Economic Affairs of Liberia. The growth rate of Liberia is lower than 23 African countries and marginally higher than 27 others.

The high population growth rate is associated with a high maternal mortality rate (49/1000 live births), which represents an estimated 20% of deaths from all causes in Liberia. For example, at the Nation's largest medical center (JFK Medical Center), 40% of all admissions to the Maternity Center were due to the complications of pregnancy, a level consistent with other hospitals around the country.

Educational System, Religion, Language, and Ethnic Division

The educational system in Liberia is of two types, formal and informal. The informal consists of the traditional "bush schools" for boys and girls while the formal comprises primary, secondary, and degree programs. The Ministry of Education is the government arm responsible for administering primary and secondary schools.

Generally, the urban areas have higher school attendance rates than the rural areas. The majority of the population in the rural areas is small farmers; literacy in these areas is not a requirement for daily life. As a result, "Western" type education is not usually adopted. Many small farmers also strongly believe that Western education will alienate their children from traditional beliefs and values and be a disruptive force within the family; hence, they are not enthusiastic about sending their children to school. It is also not uncommon for parents to allow the male child to go off to another town to school while the female child remains home under the guidance of her mother.

The "bush schools" are seen among every ethnic groups in Liberia. The *Poro* for boys and *Sande* for girls, like all schools, prepare the students for their duties in adulthood. After graduation, these bush schools confer the status of membership in the tribe; they could be used to promote economic and social development.

The beliefs discussed above probably account for the prevailing low level of literacy, particularly among women. Based on data from the 1984 Census, only 34% of the men and 17% of the females aged 10 years and over were able to read and write English. This, however, is a slight improvement over the 1974 Census figures which showed that only 30% of males and 12% of females were literate.

Moreover, there was an improvement in the attendance rates of the school-aged population from 1974 to 1984. In 1974, about 26% of the school-aged population was enrolled in school—35% of males and 17% of females— whereas by 1984, the rates had almost doubled, to about 46% of the school-aged population attending school. The differential by sex also narrowed, with 57% of males and 34% of females attending school.

There are about 28 tribes or ethnic groups in Liberia, each speaking its own dialect. The six main tribes are the Mandingo, the Kissi, the Gola, the Kpelle, the Kru, and Grebo. The largest tribe is the Kpelle. English is, however, the official language of the country.

Liberia is predominantly a Christian nation. Based on data from the 1984 Census, about 69% of the population are Christian, 14% are Muslim, and the remaining 18% belong to the category "Other or No Religion." The distribution by ethnic affiliation shows that the Kpelle, Bassa, Grebo, Kru, and Gio tribes are predominantly Christians, while the Mandingo, Vai, and Gola ethnic groups are predominantly Muslim.

Health Priorities and Programs

The Ministry of Health and Social Welfare is responsible for meeting the health and social welfare needs of the Liberian citizenry by providing a viable health care delivery system which will permeate every urban and rural community of Liberia. As will be discussed later, the health system is a centralized structure with health offices and major health supplies based in the capital, Monrovia. Over the last decade, the government of Liberia has gradually shifted from the costly curative, intensive programs of the 1970s to cost-effective, preventive-oriented primary health care programs.

The government has a health policy to care for all people through a National Health Delivery System. This system is designed to provide, in a complementary manner, preventive and curative health services throughout the country. Particular emphasis is placed on maternal and child services, environmental sanitation, immunization, and health education. The goal of the government, however, was to extend health coverage for the population from 35 % of the population to 90 % by the year 2000, at an annual rate of 3 %. It is obvious that this goal will not be realized as the health care system has been destroyed by the civil war over the last three years.

In the 1980s the government initiated the Southeast Region Primary Health Care (SER/PHC) Project, a USAID-funded program focused on two southeastern counties in Liberia. Among other things, the SER/PHC project aims at decreasing infant mortality, increasing immunization coverage of young children, educating mothers about oral rehydration therapy for diarrhea, increasing contraceptive prevalence rate, and increasing the number of deliveries by trained health workers. Its immunization efforts are aimed at combating the six major childhood diseases: measles, tetanus, poliomyelitis, tuberculosis, whooping cough, and diphtheria.

Health conditions in Liberia have been improving over the last 20 years. Life expectancy, for instance has risen, while the supply of physicians and of hospital beds has improved in relation to the size of the population. Nevertheless, the Ministry of Planning and Economic Affairs reported in 1988 that only about 35 % of Liberia's population has access to any form of modern medical services. In 1980, the total number of health facilities included 58 hospitals and health centers and 310 health posts and clinics.

DEMOGRAPHIC, SOCIOECONOMIC, AND HEALTH STATUS OF THE LIBERIAN POPULATION

Population Trends and Maternal Health

The maternal rate of increase for 1987 was 3.1%, which according to the U.S. Bureau of Census, World Population Profile, will result in a 46% increase in total population to 3.604 million by the year 2000. By comparison with other Sub-Saharan African countries, Liberia's rate of growth is the same or lower than 23 other countries including Kenya (4.2%). The associated total fertility rate is 6.7 children (Demographic and Health Survey, 1986, Bureau of Statistics, Ministry of Planning and Economic Affairs). The significance is not only demographic, e.g., increase in women of reproductive age, but the major risk of maternal and infant mortality associated with pregnancy.

Maternal mortality for Liberia in 1980, as quoted in the 1988 World Development Report, was 173/100,000 live births. The rate is not consistent with known hospital experience in Liberia and merits confirmation. Given the efforts made by the public and private Liberian health systems to introduce basic principles of modern midwifery practice at all levels, including Traditional Birth Attendants (TBAs), it would by useful to make a special effort to obtain improved national data on maternal mortality.

Maternal morbidity is also a major problem in Liberia. For example, the risk of pregnancy as illustrated in the JFK Medical Center 1986 maternal morbidity showed that almost 40% of all admissions to the maternity hospital were for complications of pregnancy. Among these complications, three types occurred in high proportions: abortions, anemia, and malaria as a chronic problem. Anemia is a consequence of multiple causes such as nutritional deficiency and repressed parasitic infection.

Population Trends and Child Health

Associated with the large proportion of women of reproductive age (46% of the total female population), high fertility, and early marriage, is a young population in which children (ages 0-14 years) comprise 43.1% of the total population (1984). In the 10-year period of 1974-1984, the recorded percentages in this age group have approximately doubled for males (23 to 43.7%) and for females (2.5-42.5%). The 0-9 age group represents approximately 75% of the total child population (UNICEF, Economic Survey of Liberia, 1985).

Demographically, the age distribution reported in these documents may not be uncommon for countries with high fertility rates and low contraceptive prevalence. The magnitude of the young population could be a clear depiction of the risk of death and illness, under Liberian conditions, from low birth weights, malnutrition, inadequate health education, and exposure to the risk of communicable disease.

Life Expectancy

The Statistical Bulletin of Liberia (1987) shows a gradual improvement in life expectancy from 53.4 years (1982) to 55 years in 1986. Grant (1991) cites an increase from 40 years in 1960 to 51 years in 1986. Information on male-to-female ratio of life expectancy was not available at the time of this document preparation. However, the life expectancy of females as a percentage of males 1987, was reported as 105.6 (Grant, 1991).

As seen in many developing countries, life expectancy has been increasing in Liberia over the years. This increase can be attributed to multiple factors. Clinical facilities and medical care are not the only factors responsible for this increase. Increased life expectancy is known to be influenced by developmental factors, particularly those which offer the populations the opportunity to protect themselves or develop physical resistance. Examples of these measures include education, nutrition, economic improvement and employment. By comparison with other Sub-Saharan countries (U.S. Bureau of Census, 1987), Liberia ranks in the top one-third (same or longer life expectancy in 18 countries, shorter expectancy in 31 countries).

Infant and Child Mortality

Available data vary widely, indicating the need for better resolution of this critical measure. Under-reporting of deaths is a component problem in many developing countries, quite aside from the efficiency of the statistical system to secure data from predominantly rural areas. However, below is a range of data illustrated by the following agencies:

1. The Ministry of Health and Social Welfare Annual Report, 1987: 50/1000 live births.

2. Demographic and Health Survey, 1986 (Ministry of Planning and Economic Affairs/Westinghouse): 44/1000 for period 1981-1986 with a decline from 192/1000 in period 1971-1975.

3. State of the World's Children, 1990 (UNICEF): 86/1000 with a decline from 153/1000 in 1960.

4. World Population Profile, 1987 (U.S. Bureau of Census): 124/1000.

The available data indicate that the precise level is not known. Accurate estimation is not an easy task, but it merits continued efforts as the measurement of infant mortality forms one of the best single indices by which to measure national health progress.

The Liberian Demographic and Health Survey indicates a decline from the high level of 275/1000 live births in the 1971-1975 period to 220/1000 in the 1981-1986. The 1985 Center for Control of Communicable Diseases (CCCD) special study using cluster sampling yielded a child mortality rate of 300/1000 in 1985. Again, we see the inconsistent figures here. Statistical methodology is all important.

Major Causes of Morbidity and Mortality in Liberia

Figures given here are based on estimates. There is poor data collection, incorrect reporting, under reporting, late reporting of monthly reports, and absence of registrars in some areas. But what is listed here offers an approximation of the underlying causes of morbidity and mortality.

According to the 1988 Annual Report of the Ministry of Health and Social Welfare, the major causes of hospitalization were malaria (18.6%), pneumonia (16.0%), anemia (12.0%), cesarean section (11.9%), abortion (12.4%), hernia (9.8%), enteritis/diarrhea (18.1%), measles (4.4%), kwashiorkor/marasmus (3.7%), motor vehicle accident (2.9%).The 10 most common outpatient diseases reported were malaria (38.5%), upper respiratory tract infection (12.5%), helminthiasis/worms (11.5%), diarrhea/enteritis (9.3%), fungus infection/ring worm (6.9%), pneumonia (5.5%), anemia (4.6%), urinary tract infection (4.6%), abscess-ulcer (3.7%), and dysentery (13.0%).

Traditional Practices and Beliefs Impacting on Health

The documented high levels of infant and child mortality, maternal mortality, and heavy burden of tropical disease are related in part to cultural beliefs and practices which are widely prevalent in Liberia. Girls are initiated into "Secret" schools between the age of 6-10 years for a duration of 2 to 3 years on the average. Boys enter the *Poro* societies often at a younger age and are taught for around 4 years. While the secret nature of these societies makes it impossible to obtain easy access to precise information, the topics for boys include tribal history, warfare, handicrafts, farming, medicine, and often more secret arts in blacksmithing and musk making. The girls are indoctrinated in household skills, farming, raising children, medicine, mat weaving, and sex education, including information on dating. Boys and girls in these societies are circumcised and subject to an oath of secrecy which places *Poro* and *Sande* leaders in a position of perceived infallibility.

How do these practices affect the health of the people? First, many people assume that communicable diseases can be treated more effectively by the traditional healer. The effect of his approach is to greatly delay the possibility of timely treatment for life-threatening illness, as in measles and severe diarrhea.

The emphasis on secrecy is believed to hinder the willingness of families to obtain early prenatal care. In Liberia, childbirth is still largely (65%) an event which is left to the traditional midwife. The Ministry of Health reported in 1988 that there were some 20,000 TBAs even though increasing numbers are receiving orientation to Western concepts. Many women still come in with complications of pregnancy. In a predominantly rural, agricultural country with strong cultural roots in traditional practices, the obstacle of attitudes serves as a major challenge to the development of improved health results on a national scale.

Liberia, being located in the tropics, may have difficulties in tackling all the health problems. For instance, one cannot change the climate or the continued prospect of insect and parasitic disease vectors. There is also no proven rapid methodology for changing traditional attitudes about health and healing. But one proposal stands out as a solution to many of these preventable diseases. One can apply the components of primary health care which may be effectively transmitted through proven technologies such as health education, environmental sanitation, protected water supply, appropriate prenatal care, family planning services, and immunization. Whether these critical services are provided through the public, nongovernmental, or private sector is not only a technical issue but one of administrative and financial design which takes into account the real options and potential for providing such services.

THE HEALTH DELIVERY SYSTEM OF LIBERIA

According to the document, Liberia Health Sector Assessment (1988), other than the extensive "Systems" of traditional medical practitioners, including traditional midwives, who are found throughout Liberia, there are five principal entities providing health services:

1.   The Ministry of Health and Social Welfare and its related semi-autonomous governmental institutions.

2.   Church-related hospitals, clinics, and training institutions.

3.   Commercial concessions (e.g., The LAMCO Hospital; Bong Mining Company Hospital; Firestone Rubber Plantations Company Hospital and The B. F. Goodrich Hospital.

4.   A growing sector of private for-profit practice which includes the private practitioner and the pharmacy and medical store networks.

5.   External private and voluntary organizations which offer health components or provide for relief services. e.g., WHO, UNESCO, UNICEF, USAID, etc.

The Ministry of Health and Social Welfare

In general, a range of services are provided by the Ministry of Health and Social Welfare (MH&SW). The specific details of services provided by the hospitals, health center, or health posts is less critical to the analysis of the health system. A review of the 1988 MH&SW Annual Report noted outreach activities from the current fixed facility in each county. These included cooperation of traditional midwives and Village Health workers at the community level; outreach teams from permanent clinics on a monthly or quarterly basis (which may include a range of preventive activities); Environmental Health Technicians (EHTs) and supervisors for Maternal and Child Health and Family Planning (MCH/FP), immunization and communicable disease control.

The structural design of the MH&SW system follows the pattern in many developing countries which emphasized curative facilities prior to the 80s. There is now a reverse as the government has realized the heavy burden of preventable disease. In many instances, government hospitals and clinics are poorly utilized, which can be considered a waste of human and financial resources. It is not surprising for clinic staff to sit in a clinic without medical supplies and medications or see fewer patients visiting these clinics.

Many of the problems seen in the hospitals, e.g., serious illness of children and complications of pregnancy which fill the hospitals, are problems which occur in communities where people live. The need for an immediate response leaves families with no immediate solution except to contact traditional healers or midwives. In fact, in many instances, the locations of hospital health centers and posts are too far from the majority of the population except those who actually live in the vicinity of a large town.

This problem is not new. So-called modern medicine is unavailable to the majority of the population in terms of convenience and accessibility. The lack of access is compounded by poor roads, heavy rainfalls, lack of transportation, and cultural traditions as discussed earlier. The MH&SW must, however, be given some credit. Prior to the 1990 civil war, the Ministry was very supportive of the strategy to extend services to the community. It is definitely to the credit and benefit of any government that assumes power in Liberia in the future to increase its reliance on the use of traditional midwives, Community Health Workers, Outreach Clinics, Village Development Committees and Community Development Committees. These are programs which merit major new attention if Liberia is serious about its National Primary Health Care Goals.

The Role of the Nongovernmental and Private Sectors

As seen in many Sub-Saharan African countries, medical missions are providing predominantly humanitarian services to the acutely ill. As early as the 1900s many health institutions, including not only schools but also clinics and hospitals, were being established by denominations such as the Lutherans, Methodists, Catholics, etc. Many of these institutions are heavily subsidized by the Liberian Government and bring in their medical supplies duty free. This has led to the sustainability of many of these hospitals which complement the work of the Ministry of Health and Social Welfare. Given the historically sustained effort by the missions (particularly in rural areas), the outlook for continued health system support by missions in the future would make it in the interest of the Government of Liberia to encourage active cooperation with these institutions.

Data on private practice in Liberia is also not clear. There is one private hospital in Monrovia, and a number of private clinics in the various counties. There may be more. Because of economic crisis in the 1980s many Liberian physicians began engaging in private practice on a part-time basis. This pattern is now being taken on by physician assistants and nurses engaging in having small clinics and medicine shop practices in the urban as well as rural areas.

Also, throughout Liberia as mentioned before, respected traditional healers continued to provide services to the population. Traditional midwives (TMs) continued to play a major role, since it is estimated that 60 to 65% of all deliveries are carried out by the TMs. Another category of people that cannot be ignored is the growing number of "black beggars" or "Quacks." These are dropouts, usually from an allied health institution, or individuals who have learned and developed some skills while working at a clinic or hospital. They offer nonprofessional and nontraditional services. Over the years, many trained health professionals have raised the questions of why these groups cannot be apprehended or eliminated since they are a threat to the population. It is not easy to do as in many instances, the "black beggars" (so-called because of the black bag they carried with their instruments and supplies) are the only ones available with common analgesics or antipyretics. This group needs to be well documented.

Government Health Policies and Strategies

In 1980, the Government of Liberia (GOL) developed a second 4-year National Socioeconomic Development Plan (1981-1985). It adopted the global consensus on "Health for All by the Year 2000." The policy language was derived almost identical to that of the World Health Assembly at Alma Ata in 1978. It stated:

Priority will be placed on the establishment of a National Primary Health Care Program designed to attain acceptable levels of health that would enable the majority of the population, especially those residing in rural areas, to lead socially and economically productive lives.

The Liberian Government at that time proposed that by the year 2000, health coverage of the population should be extended from 35 to 90%. The government strategy was to increase the per capita governmental health expenditure from $13.2 in 1979/80 to $25 by 1985. Implementation of the national PHC strategy was seriously affected by economic constraints and the political events of 1980. The long-lasting civil war will also make it difficult, if not impossible, to implement this plan.

From a policy analysis viewpoint, the government should be credited for declaring the PHC policy. This policy was an attempt to shift the balance of effort to the population majority and to obtain social equity and better distribution of limited resources. The economic reality calls for a redistribution of resources in order to achieve any reasonable progress towards providing minimal health services for the majority.

In the 1980s there were budget crises, an issue not new to many African countries as they owe the IMF and World Bank along with Western countries huge debts. The MH&SW policy also was to allocate 80% of the budget to the current hospitals and fixed facility infrastructure. Over the years, the entire health infrastructure has been slowly deteriorating and the attempts to extend health services at the periphery are limited to the few cooperative projects which the government has undertaken with external financial and technical resources. For instance, the strategies for implementing immunization programs with the Center for Control of Communicable Disease (CCCD) and the Expanded Program of Immunization (EPI), are working and coverage is increasing. But can it be sustained? The risk is that in the long term it cannot be sustained without a Liberian plan to be self-supporting.

FINANCING OF THE HEALTH SECTOR

Government Budget for the Ministry of Health and Social Welfare

The agency responsible for planning, developing, and implementing guidelines and procedures for the formulation and management of the budget is the Bureau of the Budget. On an annual basis the Bureau reviews the amount of expected revenue of the GOL and determines the budget ceiling for each ministry or agency of government. At the time the ceiling is determined there is no formal procedure whereby the ministries and agencies affected are involved. After the ceiling has been issued each has the opportunity to develop and plan its programs around the budget ceiling. The budget for the Ministry of Health and Social Welfare is developed in this manner each year.

What are the problems with this procedure? The current procedure does not provide any flexibility for the ministry to present an alternative proposal which might increase its budget allocation or even to justify the amount allocated. This process needs to be modified. It would be a good idea for each ministry or agency to present a preliminary budget to the bureau for review. It could then be reviewed in line with expected income of the GOL and each should be scheduled for a budget hearing. After the budget has been reviewed and justified, the final budget of each ministry or agency can then be determined.

The GOL provides budgetary support to health care sector through the MH&SW and the JFK Medical Center. Although the JFK Medical Center is administratively autonomous from the MH&SW, the budgetary support given to it by the GOL is considered as part of the overall GOL support of the health sector. According to the Economic Recovery Program 1986-1989, the financial support to the health sector by the GOL has changed considerably over the past years. The recurrent health budget rose from $14.9 million in 1977-78 to $30.9 million in 1981-82, and then fell to a low of $18.8 million in 1988.

In a depressed economic situation as seen in Liberia, it becomes imperative that the health sector be allowed to obtain the highest possible value for its money. This can be achieved only by reprogramming available resources into activities which will bring about the best overall results in the priority curative and preventive areas without exceeding the ability of the public and private sector to provide health costs. Reprogramming, however, calls for redesign of the service system consistent with limited resources.

Fee-for-Service Systems

Prior to 1986 the GOL had a policy of very low or no cost to the public for health services at its facilities. But as the overall GOL and health sector budget began to decline, it became increasingly difficult for the GOL to provide the funding support necessary for such a policy. In 1985, the president gave his approval to a policy to decentralize the health systems and to implement "Fee-for-Service" (FFS) and "Revolving Drug Fund" (RDF) systems at the county level.

The FFS is a procedure whereby patients pay the clinician, health worker, or facility a specified amount of money for the medical services. In conjunction with this, the RDF system permits patients to pay for the drugs received. The monies collected are put aside for the replenishment of drugs. The purpose of the FFS is to recover as much as possible the non-salary recurrent cost of each facility. At the health center/health post level, the amounts needed to recover these costs might be relatively low; however, at the hospital level these amounts can be substantial. At the hospital level the FFS monies are usually used to offset the general operating costs of the hospital.

Revolving Drug Fund Systems

The RDF systems in government hospitals began at the same time as the FFS systems. These systems were necessitated as a result of the inability of the GOL to provide drugs to its facilities from 1983-1986. Despite the existence of a National Medical Supply Depot (NMSD), it had large uncollectible accounts receivable and could not replenish drug stocks. This created a situation where government hospitals and clinics had no drugs and medical supplies to treat patients.

In an effort to alleviate the problem mentioned above, the NMSD was dissolved and the National Drug Service (NDS) established. This service procures drugs through the International Dispensary Association and other budget suppliers of bulk drugs. At the county level, RDFs are established in most cases by the hospital, community, and a donor. These systems provide a central location where the health centers and posts can purchase the drugs and medical supplies needed for their facilities without going to the capital or a local retailer. Because RDFs have the potential to generate cash by the sale of drugs to patients or to the retail market, close supervision of each health center/post is essential.

Foreign Exchange Needs

The health sector of Liberia, as in many other developing countries, has had increasing difficulty obtaining foreign exchange to purchase the necessary drugs for the system. The continued credibility of the government's curative system is dependent on the availability of drugs, particularly in the counties. In the absence of a Liberian pharmaceutical industry, medicines must be purchased abroad. The World Health Organization (WHO) has furnished countries with a list of medicines, or "formulary" known as essential drugs. These are advocated by WHO as low-cost drugs.

The dependency on drug availability is so important to the MH&SW system that failure to procure drugs cripples the system. The problem is not the availability of cash in Liberian dollars collected from patients but the conversion of this cash into foreign exchange for the required purchases.

The functioning of critical field demonstration programs such as the South Eastern Region Primary Health Care (SER/PHC) would deteriorate rapidly without the availability of drugs. The MH&SW should therefore undertake a study of alternative sources for foreign exchange (commercial sources, missions, UNICEF, concessions) to determine practical availability and the effect of cost increases to the consumer. The issue is to determine if consumers would find it acceptable to pay a small increase in costs for essential drugs which are already inexpensive.

External Technical and Financial Cooperation

According to the 1986 edition of the Geographic Distribution of Financial Flows to Developing Countries, there are about 21 bilateral and multilateral sources cooperating in Liberia. The Ministry of Health and Social Welfare cites at least 11 external sources which have cooperated with the GOL in health and development. Some of these include cooperation with the governments of Japan, Germany, China, and the Netherlands. Other agencies include UMFPA, UNICEF, WHO, and USAID. Too much reliance on single sources, such as USAID, may be inappropriate because of the historical growth of development among other members of the industrialized nations.

The MH&SW should establish a unit which is trained and oriented in the mobilization of external financing for health. Lessons can be learned from PAHO Guidelines for external financial planning. The MH&SW should do all it can to attract external concessional financing for health.

HEALTH MANPOWER OF LIBERIA

Development of Health Manpower

Trained health manpower is employed by both the private and public sector. The GOL hospitals, mission hospitals, and private concession hospitals all play key roles in the employment process. Trained health manpower refers to physicians, PAs, pharmacists, RNs, CMs, LPNs, nurse's aides, EHTs, and other preventive health personnel.

Without a detailed study of each hospital it is not possible to determine if staffs are appropriate for the mix of patients or for the level of care provided. An important factor in making such a determination is the degree to which caretakers, family, and students provide patient care.

There are rural/urban staffing disproportions, low utilization rates in hospitals and clinics, and the limitation of outreach services by existing facilities. The pattern reflects a dysfunctionality of deployment which is partly a consequence of the budget constraints over the years. The situation also affects the orientation of training, which is dominantly curative, the absence of career structures or incentives, and the loss of personnel from the government rolls, particularly nurses.

In the current situation, manpower issues cannot be limited to numbers, qualifications, and training resources but must include the relationship of manpower to governmental policy and financial planning. As long as the government adheres to its policy of extending essential health care to the population majority through the PHC approach, manpower issues should be seen through the same lens. Liberia cannot now afford to adequately support its current level of manpower. The existing manpower also is not yet oriented to the official policy goals of the MH&SW.

According to the 1988 Annual Report of the MH&SW, the estimated total number of health personnel in Liberia in public and private categories is 5,056. This includes 237 physicians (4.7%); 556 professional nurses and midwives, all levels (13%); 2,782 traditional midwives (55%); and 1,381 other supporting personnel (27.3%). The ratio of physician per population is 1:10,126. According to a UNICEF report, this is equal or better than one-third of Sub-Saharan countries, including Kenya. However, as seen in other African countries, the maldistribution of physicians favors the urban areas. It is estimated that 75% of Liberia's physicians are in Monrovia (Liberia's capital). Monrovia, according to varying estimates, contains 25% of the total population.

At the current stage of Liberia's health development, the physician is not the most effective or appropriate professional category to meet the health objectives of Liberia in terms of communicable disease reduction, prenatal care, environmental sanitation, or development of health services in widely distributed rural areas. To have a major impact on the reduction of primary causes of illness and death, it is more appropriate to retrain and redeploy personnel to take on the task of serving the community. Nurses could be trained in the area of PHC to reach out to the community. However, major inequalities apply to nurses as well: Almost half of all professional nurses are located in Monrovia.

Training of Health Manpower

Health manpower is trained at two universities, a National Institute of Medical Arts, and four hospital-based training programs at two universities. These institutions train for the following professions: physicians, pharmacists, professional nurses, environmental health technicians, RN/midwives, laboratory assistants/technicians, physician assistants, practical nurses, and certified midwives. Dental assistants and X-ray technicians have in the past been trained in Liberia, but due to lack of funds in the 1980s, these programs have become inactive.

Training programs in Liberia have been affected by the same problems of budget constraints that adversely influence the entire health sector. With the diversity of training institutions, it is difficult to generalize. Basic to this analysis is the assumption that training cannot be separated from the demand for personnel. Given budget constraints, the factors of redundancies, shortages, maldistribution, and inappropriate mix of health personnel should be considered in training objectives. New staffing models which reflect more realistic utilization by facility and the shift in emphasis towards outreach with PHC should serve as the guidance for restructuring national programs.

Registration of Trained Health Workers

Liberia registers (licenses or certifies) the following health workers: physicians, pharmacists, dentists, RNs, nurse midwives, practical nurses, nurse aide, midwives, operating room technicians, and traditional midwives. Liberia maintains an established structure of registration which should be continued, improved, and enforced. The problem, however, is that registration as a condition of employment is not uniformly monitored and enforced. Registration of health professionals is very important to maintaining standards of professional performance and the quality of health care. It is also an excellent source of data on trained health care workers in Liberia. Steps should be taken to require that all health workers be registered and that they maintain their registration as a condition of employment.

HEALTH SERVICE UTILIZATION

There is maldistrubution of health facilities in Liberia. Distance plays a major role in when or how people seek care. This is not meant to downplay the importance of traditional beliefs and attitudes that affect health care-seeking patterns.

Several studies have determined that physical proximity is an important factor in accessibility and utilization of health care resources. Closeness to a particular doctor or facility is one of the main reasons for using that resource. The importance of distance seems obvious, but unfortunately, it has often been ignored in planning decisions. It would be interesting to examine what happens to the distance people have to travel to when the hospital nearest them closes. The health care provider-client link weakens as distance increases. The distance traveled to hospitals is also affected by other important factors such as type and severity of illness. Because of the distance, it is not uncommon for a pregnant woman to arrive in the emergency room of a hospital in Liberia fully dilated or to have delivered hours ago and begun hemorrhaging.

The discussion of distance could be viewed from different perspectives. Meade (1988), discussed distance measures which are applicable to the Liberian settling. These include road distance-which takes into account the actual or supposed route taken from home to the practitioner. This measure can be weighted by road quality. As discussed earlier, road quality in many parts of Liberia is very poor as in many other Sub-Saharan countries. The quality of the road, for example, is a key factor leading to complications of some illnesses e.g. premature labor, spontaneous abortion, etc. Other forms of distances are time distance and mobility distance. Many clients have to walk for days to reach a health post, at times only to be told that there is not any help or medication available. When that client becomes ill on the second occasion, he/she chooses going to her rice farm rather than to waste time repeating the entire process.

Some important distance measures that do not involve distance in geographic sense are sociocultural distances. Social distance is the gap between consumer and provider in terms such as social status or illness beliefs. Economic distance is the ability to pay for services. These sociocultural distance measures can be used in accessibility and utilization studies. While citizens of Liberia do not have to deal with racial prejudice as seen in some other countries, there is the factor of "class" and "status" which cannot be ignored.

Distance is not the only factor leading to underutilization of health services in Liberia. In Liberia, as in many developing countries, facilities within a few miles of most of the population may be rarely used because their quality is poor. Therefore, distance should be considered in relation to other variables.

In Liberia, except in counties targeted by the South Eastern Region Primary Health Care Project (SER/PHC), staffing is far from adequate. The rapport between clinics and their surrounding communities is poor or non-existent. Services are delivered in an unplanned manner at health posts due to deficient skills, absence of equipment and shortage of supplies. Finally, staff morale is low as a in consequence.

The largest hospitals, called referral hospitals (e.g., JFK Memorial and Phebe Hospitals), consist of medical specialist and dentist and intensive care facilities along with specialized equipment appropriate to such services. Ministry of Health and Social Welfare hospitals are located at the county seats and in Monrovia. Inpatient care is therefore far removed from the rural areas, a situation which is underscored by poor roads and lack of transportation for the referral of patients.

Besides catering to inpatients, hospitals provide large outpatient departments offering special services such as prenatal care, family planning, well-baby care, medical consultation and immunization. Most cases seen in hospitals are emergency admissions. Many patients succumb during the journey to the hospital. What is especially noteworthy is that among women of childbearing age and children the high hospital fatality rates encountered reflect both delay in seeking help and ill-advised self-medication.

Mid-level care available closer to communities would be more appropriate than the present situation, where beds are concentrated in hospitals with low utilization rates in county seats. Many conditions which are seen in rural clinics need treatment or care immediately. Among children, examples include cases of dehydration, pneumonia, meningitis, malaria, and other childhood communicable diseases such as measles and whooping cough. For these problems, better use could be made of the holding beds already located at some clinics. Often a life-saving course of therapy can be administered in this setting; in other cases efforts can be made to stabilize the patients until suitable means of referral can be found.

As noted earlier, the serious illness of children and the complications of pregnancy which fill the hospitals are problems which occur in the communities in which people live. The need for an immediate response leaves families with no solution except to contact traditional healers or midwives. In effect, the locations of hospitals, centers and posts are too far from the majority of the population, except those who actually live in the vicinity or a large town. The best way to resolve this problem is through primary health care activities in which PHC workers will be available to the people in the community.

Another possibility is the integration of traditional medicine and modern medicine. In many countries, traditional (professional and non-professional) and biomedicine coexist. But in most instances there is little cooperation between these two systems.

Several policy options are open to those in charge of the health delivery system in Liberia—which has both traditional and modern components. Some policy makers may suggest that traditional medicine be made illegal. This, however, will not be a realistic approach. In Nigeria and Ghana, legislation has been passed to license traditional healers. However, the license is no guarantee of good quality traditional practices. Another approach, which is supported by the World Health Organization (WHO), is to gradually increase cooperation between modern and traditional practitioners. It must be done intelligently. There is an advantage of medical pluralism which provides diversity and maturity. In my opinion this is the only viable option. From experience, no matter how much health education is given to our clients, they are still likely to seek the traditional healer for some ailments, especially ones that seem difficult to diagnose or cure in the hospital.

If integration of modern medicine with traditional medicine is proposed for the Liberian health care system, how is this process going to be implemented? The first step is to look critically at the strengths and weaknesses of both systems. In Western medicine, there have been many discoveries. For example, vaccines, antibiotics and various drugs were developed after World War II which led to a decrease in morbidity and mortality around the world. Western medicine can also boast of advances in surgical techniques and effective use of technology.

However, the biomedical model emphasizes cure and expensive technology. In areas like Liberia where prevention would solve far more health problems and where people are poor, this model is inappropriate. In Liberia, as in many other

Sub-Saharan countries, doctors and other health care professionals including nurses, are trained based on the biomedical model, either in their countries or abroad. Health care workers are not trained to deal with local health problems. They know very little abut the cultural, political, and economic environments in which disease is experienced and help sought. Indigenous Liberian doctors trained in Western medicine often are reluctant to serve outside Monrovia (capital of Liberia). Some leave the country for more lucrative practices in industrialized countries, where they can use the technology they have studied. The issue of "brain drain" of health manpower in Liberia will be discussed later. The trend has been increased by the civil war in Liberia.

Another health resource factor in Liberia is that those who enter medical college or study medicine are usually from families of the upper class or so-called elite groups. Thus, the elite control the Ministry of Health and the Health Care System and they also perpetuate the hegemony of biomedicine. They are also not aware of what the average citizen faces when seeking health. They are far removed from the general population by dressing, gestures, attitudes, and behavior. As a result, building a prestigious teaching hospital like the JFK Medical Center in Monrovia took precedence over providing a minimum level of health care for all the people of Liberia.

Why support traditional medicine? The main positive quality of traditional medicine is that it is part of the people it serves. Traditional healers convey social and psychological benefits through sympathy for a patient's beliefs and feelings. Traditional medicine is holistic in nature. It treats body and mind and attempts to integrate the person, society, and physical environment. It must be noted that some of the drugs developed by traditional healers over many centuries are very effective. Traditional healers in Liberia such as bonesetters and TBAs cannot be ignored.

What, then, are some criticisms of traditional medicine? Indigenous healers have been criticized for several possible shortcomings. Many of their herbs may be ineffective, and cures are often based on trial and error. Pharmacologists may also argue that ignorance of proper drug dosage can be dangerous. Witchcraft and sorcery practices are potentially harmful. While it is no secret that Western medicines are expensive, indigenous healers have also been known to have their eyes on the marketplace. Many of their healings that were done free or for very little are now driven by the economy. Both systems, however, attract quacks.

Successful integration of modern and traditional practice is most likely if it follows the goals of primary health care. As stated in the Alma Ata Proceedings, these goals include emphasis on self-reliance and decision making at the local level, the use of paramedical personnel for lower levels of care, appropriate technology, geographic, financial, cultural, and functional accessibility to prevention and treatment.

EDUCATIONAL ACHIEVEMENT FOR WOMEN

All around the world people are advocating increases in woman's status. One way to confer said status is through equal opportunity for educational achievement. If a woman is educated, an entire generation has been educated—especially in societies where the woman bears the greater bulk of the responsibilities. There is no doubt that progress has been made over the years to provide education to women in Liberia; however, there is still a huge gap. Due to the lack of information it will be impossible to state exactly the male/female ratios at different levels of school in Liberia or ratio of males/females in fields of advanced study and training. Reports given here will only be estimates based on several sources.

According to the 1984 Census (the latest Census), only 34% of men and 17% of women aged 10 years and over were able to read and write English. It was also reported that in 1974 about 26% of the school-aged population were males and 17% females. In 1984, the rates increased to 46% of school-aged attending school. The differential for sex also narrowed, with 57% of males and 34% of females attending school. This increase was probably due to the National Socioeconomic Development Plan (1976-1980) which made "universal basic education" an explicit development objective. It must be noted that universal education even at the primary level is yet not attained despite a public school law which was passed in 1839, and revised in 1912 promulgating compulsory education in Liberia.

The pattern of colonization and Western ideology promoted in Liberia and other Sub-Saharan countries helped to create the atmosphere for current gaps between men and women. Liberia was not actually colonized as other African countries, but being on the coast of the Atlantic Ocean there were several European countries (e.g., Great Britain, Portugal, and Spain) that traded in Liberia. The freed slaves who arrived from the United States also brought suppressive ideologies. There were infiltration of missionaries of different denominations in Liberia including Catholic, Lutheran, Baptist, Methodist, and almost any form of Christian denomination seen in the U.S.A.

The generation of free slaves in Liberia are commonly known as Americo-Liberians. These are the elite groups that chose to build their own institutions and separate themselves from the indigenous population. As mentioned previously, this minority group ruled for centuries and could be seen as a direct replication of oppression they encountered while in slavery in the U.S.A. As people in leadership, most of the policies, including educational policies, were dictated by them. Many of these polices were also heavily directed to the Americo-Liberian population and not to the entire population. It was difficult for an indigenous person to attend a good school, i.e., private school. Government supported free education at the primary level, but many of the government schools were not good academically. It was not uncommon for the Americo-Liberian to send his/

her child to school abroad, either to the U.S.A or to Europe. The interest, therefore, in supporting the local schools was nonexistent.

Women were regarded in the Liberian culture as being fit only for functioning as a housewife and not capable of gaining higher education. Few girls were given the opportunities to gain higher education by the missionaries. The missionaries came in with their own ideas on how girls should be educated. The idea was to make them wonderful wives and great mothers. A girl is usually deprived from attending school in the same county where she gets pregnant. She must travel to another county if she wants to continue her education. According to the Ministry of Education officials, this is done to set an example for other students. Children enter school very late in Liberia although the trend is now changing. It is not uncommon to find a 14 or 16-year-old girl still in the 4th or 5th grade. Mothers are more comfortable with their sons going to school than their daughters. Even with the government compulsory education policy for all children to be sent to school, many parents still choose not to send their daughters to school. This creates an enormous problem as she reaches the stage of maturity while still being in the elementary school. With the unavailability of contraceptives and abortion being illegal, when a teenager gets pregnant, she is left with no other option but to face the consequences of expulsion from school. The boy who impregnated her is allowed to continue school and thereby increases the chances for males to complete secondary school on time and go on for further education.

These policies are not really seen in universities. But while girls are able to attend primary schools in greater numbers, by the time the group gets to the universities, the ratio of girls to boys is very low. Many females have become pregnant and forced to drop out of school to support their child. At the university levels, there are entrance examinations taken before a student is admitted. That student also has to produce his/her National Exam Certificate issued by the Government through the West African Examination Council. Despite the lack of statistical data, only a few girls are accepted to the universities. It is not uncommon for entrance exam proctors to demand bribes or harass the girls before they are admitted. In essence, a female who enters college has really overcome many barriers that males did not have when they pursued further education.

One issue that existed in the earlier days was the policy of forced marriage instituted by the church and missionaries. It was a common practice until recently to demand that a boy marry the girl he impregnated. In many instances, they were only teenagers, they were not experienced, and had no education or profession or any kind of financial base. Who suffered more from such policies? It was the girl since on many occasions, the boy eventually left her anyway.

The ratio of males/females in the fields of advanced degrees and training is not known. However, there is an increasing number of women seeking advanced degrees abroad. According to the Human Development Report, (1992), third level students abroad (as a percentage of those at home) seeking higher education between 1987-1988 was 18.0%. Efforts are needed on the part of the government or those agencies responsible for manpower development in Liberia to recruit more women for advanced training in areas relevant to the development of Liberia.

SOCIOECONOMIC STATUS OF WOMEN IN LIBERIA

Economic output normally increases as capacity investment increases and as more workers join the labor force. But increases in productivity also play an important part. Productivity in Liberia is small as is true in many other developing countries. Generally, productivity increases have been attributed to several factors: technical innovation, a healthier and more advanced skilled work force or a more vigorous entrepreneurial spirit. All these are usually the reward for investing in education and health, building up the country's "human capital."

In developed as well in developing countries there is usually a disparity in the degree of equality of wealth of a country or the number of women in the labor force and type of occupation. Estimates given here are based on the Human Development Report, 1992. For Liberia, it was reported that the labor force as a percentage of the total population between 1988-1990 was 36.2%. And women in the labor force, as a percent of the total labor force for 1988-1990, was 30.6%. The statistics may be inaccurate since the percentage of males educated in Liberia is greater than females. Women play a major role in agriculture in Liberia as well as in other Sub-Saharan Countries. They work hard in fields to bring food to the tables for their families. It is also reported in the Human Development Report (1992) that in 1965, 79.0% of the labor force was involved in agriculture in Liberia and between 1986-1989 the figure dropped to 74.4%.

The percentage of the population involved in agriculture may be underestimated in the Human Development Report. It is clear that most Liberians are subsistence farmers and many grow rice, cocoa, coffee, and rubber. Rice is the staple food for most Liberians. Because of the lack of technology, rice is still not grown on a large scale. Most of what is grown is also taken to the market for sale to get money for other needed goods. The country therefore relies heavily on imported rice from abroad.

The percent of the labor force in industry and service is low. Liberia has several natural resources such as gold, diamond, and iron ore. These products are being mined by expatriates. The Human Development Report (1992) cites 10% of the population involved in industrial work in 1965. This number decreased to 9.4% between 1986-1989. In the area of service work, the percent of the labor force involved was 11% and it increased to 16.4% between 1986-1989. With depreciating prices for iron ore and rubber, most of the companies began to close in the 1980s. As the unemployment rate increased, many Liberians had no choice but to turn to the service industry.

What constitutes the "working population" in Liberia is not clear. The 1984 Population and Housing Census (the latest census) does not define the concept either. The census, however, examines working population 10 years and over and showed an increase between 1974-1984 greater than between the 1962 and 1974 period. There was an increment of nearly 5.5% in the latter intercensual period as compared to 5% in the former period. Table 2-1 presents the working population 10 years and over in Liberia by year and by sex.

Table 2-1. Working Population 10 Years and Over in Liberia

Year	Males	Females
	All Industry	
1984	388,323	281,007
1974	316,849	116,023
1964	263,560	148,234
	Agriculture	
1984	234,274	234,401
1974	206,196	97,499
1962	185,998	138,260

Source: Summary Population Results—1984 Population and Housing Census, Republic of Liberia.

The increase in working population was shared differently by the sexes. It was reported in the 1984 census that males increased by 71,474 between 1974 and 1984. In the case of females, there was an increase of 164,984 between 1974 and 1984. Between 1962 and 1974, the number of female workers was significantly less at 32,211. Further examination of the differential in the working population shows a substantial increase among female agricultural workers between the intercensual period of 1974 and 1984. What, then, is responsible for the sudden increase in female workers? Possible reasons for this rapid increase experienced by female agricultural workers include the following: 1) An under enumeration of female agricultural workers in the 1974 census, 2) differential under enumeration and over enumeration bias in all three censuses, and 3) females' neglecting schooling and engaging in more farming activities during 1984. The third rationale is less plausible due to increasing evidence that there has been an increase in the number of literate females in Liberia.

An overview of the working pattern reveals a similar trend as seen in Table 2-1. In 1984, 46.6% of the population age 10 years and over was classified as working people compared to rates of 41.2 and 57.4% in 1974 and 1962 respectively. Among males, the data show some decline from 74.6 in 1962 to 59.9 in 1974 and finally to 53.4% in 1984. Similar fluctuating trend is shown among the working population of females, from 40.7% in 1962 to 22.2% in 1974 and 39.6% in 1984. The current pattern cannot be determined. The next census was to be held in 1990 but was not done because of the civil war. There are no laws that ban women from owning a property. If a female has sufficient capital, she can purchase a piece of land, build and a own house or own or operate a business. The ownership of land is usually passed on from one generation to the next. However, in many traditional families, it is not uncommon for the father to give the property to the male child. As in many other cultures, there is still the perception that women are weak and will not be able to care for or maintain family order where a father dies. This pattern is changing in households without a male child the girl inherits the property.

There is now increasing number of single female households. Many are single because of divorce and others because of an early death of their husband. Single female households receive help in raising their children from extended family members. When a female is dropped from secondary school or college she often is able to continue her education due to the willingness of her mother or other relatives to care for her children, usually at no cost while she is away at school often in a distant town or city.

FAMILY STRUCTURE

Current Marital Status

Childbearing in Liberia takes place within prescribed and relatively stable marital unions. It is essential to study the patterns of marriage in all the Liberian ethnic groups in order to better understand fertility patterns in Liberia. The Liberian Demographic and Health Survey (LDHS) (1986), defines marriage loosely to include any legal or customary union of a man and a woman as husband and wife, as well as other stable cohabitation, such as a man and a woman living together and having sexual relations without any legal or customary binding.

In a heterogenous culture such as Liberia, the definition above is appropriate for most groups. It is not uncommon to hear a man or a woman call each other husband and wife after living together for three or more years. Forced marriage exists today among some Liberian ethnic groups but to a lesser degree. Previously a girl was considered rebellious if she refused to marry the man selected for her by her parents. Nowadays, forced marriage ceremonies could be halted if a girl refuses to accept the man. In the past, inter-tribal marriage was very low or non-existent among many ethnic groups but this pattern is changing rapidly. The Mandingo tribe who are Moslems strongly discourage their children from marrying a person from a different ethnic group. Based on the LDHS definition of marriage, it was reported that one out of every five respondent in the LDHS had never been married, 67% were currently married, while 11% were either widowed, divorced, separated or no longer living together. Table 2-2 presents the percent distribution of women by current marital status for 1986.

Table 2-2. Percent Distribution of Women by Marital Status and Age in 1986.

Age	Never Married	Married	Living Together	Widowed	Divorced	Not Living Together	Weighted Number
15-19	64.0	9.7	22.0	0.4	1.4	2.5	1,137
20-24	27.7	20.2	45.3	0.1	2.5	7.1	1,030
25-29	7.9	34.2	45.1	0.6	3.2	9.0	1,081
30-34	6.2	38.3	43.5	1.7	3.5	6.8	658
35-39	1.2	42.4	43.1	2.4	4.5	6.4	626
40-44	1.7	40.3	39.7	6.6	4.4	7.3	327
45-49	0.5	51.0	30.8	6.2	5.7	5.8	380
All Ages	21.4	29.2	38.3	1.6	3.1	6.3	5,239

Source: Demographic and Health Survey of Liberia, 1986. Bureau of Statistics, Ministry of Planning and Economic Affairs, 1988.

The table above shows the variations in marital status by current age of the LDHS respondents. According to the table, the proportion of women who have never married decreases substantially with increasing age. At age 15-19 the never married proportion is 6% but decreases to about 1% by age 35. This is not an unusual pattern. The proportion of women reported as living together is considerably higher in each age group than compared to those legally married. The extent of widowerhood is relatively small, particularly in the younger age groups, 15-19 through 30-34 years. Similarly, the proportion of women divorced is small and increases with age. It would be interesting to compute the LDHS data on nuptiality with other sources of data in order to assess trends in marriage patterns and to evaluate the quality of data. The age at marriage has been rising.

POLYGYNY AND ITS IMPLICATIONS

The LDHS Data revealed that 38% of women in the study were in polygamous unions. However, there are no other sources of demographic information to which these data can be compared to detect any trend over time. The

LDHS data show that the prevalence of polygynous unions in Liberia increases slightly with the age of the women. Could it be that the practice is gradually eroding? Or do these data reflect the fact that as women get older, their husbands are more likely to take second wives.

According to the LDHS (1988), polygyny is more common in rural Liberia (43% of currently married women) than in the urban areas (30%). The rate is higher in rural Liberia because of their way of living. In rural Liberia people are predominately farmers. Many men want more wives to enhance their political and economic status and to satisfy their desire for children. The more wives a man has, the stronger he is considered, the larger his farm (each wife cultivates a plot of land), and the greater the number of children.

The desire for children is one of the ultimate goals of most Liberian unions; even in monogamous unions, many men have children outside marriage by their girlfriends. It may be shocking to see the high rate of polygyny in urban areas. One would expect that life in an urban area is more competitive and the cost of living is much higher than in rural areas. Most urban residents are primarily engaged in economic activities apart from farming, thus eliminating the need for wives to cultivate plots of land. Polygyny is inversely related to educational attainments. From observations, uneducated women are more likely to be polygynous than women who have attained secondary or higher levels of education. Education and urban residence are highly correlated and it is difficult to separate the effects of the two variables on polygyny.

A higher proportion (51%) of Muslim women than Christian (34%) are in polygamous unions. Although polygyny is contrary to the Christian religion, religious groups in Liberia still find it difficult convincing individuals to be monogamous. Polygynous marital unions are found among 32% of women in other or traditional religions and 41% percent of women who have no religious affiliation. Differences in the extent of polygyny by tribal groups range from a high of 57% among the Mandingo to a low of 24% among the Gola tribe (LDHS Gola Tribe, 1986). In addition to its association with a lower status for women, polygyny carries some health implications such as STDs and AIDS. However, it would be inappropriate to target only those with polygynous relationships. Many other groups to target for AIDS and STDs prevention include prostitutes and those who practice "silent polygyny," i.e., they claim to be in a monogamous relationship but are constantly cheating on their spouses.

According to the WHO reports of AIDS cases reported by African countries, there were only two cases reported in Liberia in 1987. It is obvious that the disease is under reported and as will be mentioned later, Liberian refugees faced a greater risk of developing the disease as they reside in nearby countries such as the Ivory Coast, Sierra Leone, and Guinea. It has been rumored that many young female Liberian refugees are becoming prostitutes on the streets of neighboring countries. Once the country returns to normal, many of these refugees will return home with the AIDS virus.

With a fatal disease such as AIDS, polygyny is definitely a risk factor, but it will take an immense effort to change a behavior that has been deep rooted in the culture for years. For the age of prevention to take hold, communication is necessary to build a societal consensus—a public code of ethics—that performing these new behaviors is the "right" way to behave. In order for most people to adopt new behaviors and maintain them, it is imperative that public opinion support the new behaviors (Lanstey and Piot, AIDS Prevention in Africa, 1990).

If the Liberian people believe that their peers as well as their family support having only one sexual partner—and the opinion of their peers and family is important to them—they will be more motivated to remain monogamous than if the reverse were true. What is important is the perceived reliance of an individual or group on the approval or disapproval of the behavior.

AGE AT FIRST UNION AND
EXPOSURE TO RISK OF PREGNANCY

Information on marriage aspect is based on the Liberian Demographic and Health Survey. Caution should be taken in interpreting any data on age in Liberia as, like many developing countries, Liberians have difficulty placing events in time.

Another factor related to about marriage age is the custom of sending girls to live in the household of their future husbands at a young age. The LDHS reported that a small proportion of women stated very young ages at marriage due to this custom. Presumably said marriages were not consummated until the girls matured.

Half (50%) of Liberian women enter into marriage before reaching the age of 18. An additional 12% are first married between the ages of 18-19 years, while 17% marry at age 20 or older. The younger women have a higher median age at first marriage urban women (18.5 years) than rural women (16.8 years). Education is also highly correlated with age at first marriage. The higher the level of education, the higher the median age at first marriage. At each age group, women with no education marry at much younger ages than women who have attended secondary school (Liberian Demographic and Health Survey, 1986).

There are differentials by ethnicity in age at marriage. The LDHS cites the median age for first marriages at (18.0). The LDHS reports indicates that the following ethnic groups—Mano, Gio, Gola, Krahn, Mandingo, and Bassa—marry earlier than women of other tribes. These are some inconsistencies which may be due to memory lapse on the part of older women who could not remember their ages at first marriages.

What does this early age at first union have to do with exposure to the risk of pregnancy? The LDHS cited 15% of women in the survey who are currently married and were pregnant. As expected, the proportion declines with increasing age, ranging from over 22% among women in age group 15-19 to only 5% among those in the 45-49 age group. Although the proportion of women exposed to conception is higher among younger women, even older women seem to have relatively high proportions of women who are susceptible to becoming pregnant. This implies that the provision of family planning services should not be limited to young women but should also be extended to older women. It should be noted that some of the women might want another child or might already be using some method of family planning.

Divorce Laws and Divorce Rates

Legally, if a couple chooses not to remain together for life, one person may file a divorce. The case is usually decided by a judge who divides any property the couples has accumulated. Divorce rates in Liberia are not high there are no definitive statistics to prove this. My remarks are based on observation and talks with some other Liberians while studying in the United States. There may be differences between the urban area where people live a more Western style of life as opposed to the rural area where people are more cohesive and traditional.

In the past, marriages were long-lasting. The Liberian people are more community oriented a family approves the marriage of a daughter after serious back ground checks are done even if it is not a pre arranged marriage. If one of the elders in that family does not approve of the wedding the ceremony is usually delayed or cancelled. Opinions of the elders in the village including close relatives are highly respected. Once the ceremony for a marriage has been held, the elders expect it to last until one of the partners dies. If there are some problems in the marriage, it is expected that the elders will sit around a table and discuss how to resolve that conflict. In almost all ethnic groups in Liberia, to divorce your partner would mean convincing your mother, father and the elders in the village that the divorce was appropriate. There must be a justifiable reason for a woman to leave her husband or for a man to leave his wife. One such reasons is usually violence against the woman in the form of physical abuse. If a man is constantly beating his wife she will be asked to leave for the compound of her relative to avoid him.

There may be some advantages and disadvantages to this process. One advantage is that the unnecessary money usually spend on divorce cases can be saved. Moreover, the settlement of complaints in a timely fashion by the relatives of both partners and other elders in the community can strengthen the bond between both families. A serious disadvantage with the Liberian approach is that a woman may be caught in a relationship where she is not happy but societal norms force her to remain in that relationship and endure torture at home. In Liberia, many complaints in addition to marriage are settled at home or by the elders in the community. It is considered selfish or inhumane to take your neighbors to court and have them pay money to the government. This is the reason for the government allowing the existence of tribal courts ran by village chiefs. The chiefs are empowered to decide a variety of cases.

Breastfeeding, Postpartum Amenorrhea, and Abstinence

The LDHS collected data on several factors other than contraception that affect the length of pregnancy intervals. These included breastfeeding amenorrhea, and sexual abstinence. The practice of breastfeeding is very common among Liberian women. Most women breastfeed their children for long periods. The mean and median duration of breastfeeding in Liberia is almost identical at 17 months. Breastfeeding diminishes significantly after this time. LDHS also reports that the average breastfeeding duration in Liberia is similar to that of other Sub-Saharan Countries, such as Benin (19 months), Cameroon, Ghana, Ivory Coast, and Senegal (18 months), and Kenya (17 months).

While most mothers in Liberia perceived breastfeeding as a traditional behavior and do breastfeed, there is an increasing group of young semi-educated women who choose not to breastfeed at all. They choose to bottle feed their children. The reasons given for not breastfeeding are, it is an old-fashioned idea and breastfeeding will cause their breasts to sag. There is also a growing perception that when a mother bottle feeds her baby with formula, she is of a higher class than other women. As a result, scarce family resources are spent on commercial formulas. This leads to an economic loss to the family and bottle feeding serves as a precursor for diarrhea and respiratory diseases, two major killers of under-5s in African and other developing countries where sanitation is poor and pure water resources are scarce.

The amenorrheic period for most women depends on their physiological condition and such factors as nutrition and length of breastfeeding. The LDHS data indicated the median duration of postpartum amenorrhea is about 8 months and the mean is about 11 months. This is reportedly similar to other Sub-Saharan countries such as Benin, Cameroon, and Ghana (12 months), and Ivory Coast and Kenya (10 months).

In Liberia as in many other Sub-Saharan countries, postpartum sexual abstinence is widely practiced. The duration is usually tied to ongoing breastfeeding which is considered essential to the health and normal development of the child. The LDHS also reported the postpartum abstinence had a median duration of 11 months. It is widely believed that while breastfeeding there should be no sex and that once sex commences, the breast milk is poison for the child and no longer good for the child. Many women including men also abide this rule. Some breastfeeding literature has shown that educated women are unlikely to breastfeed for long durations, primarily due to greater participation in the labor force. There is a changing trend in the U.S.A. with women of high socioeconomic status now choosing to breastfeed while women of low socioeconomic status have declining breastfeeding patterns. The LDHS reported that women with secondary or higher education breastfed their children for an average of only 10 months, as compared to 17 months for women with primary education and 19 months for women with no education.

SEXUALITY, CONTRACEPTIVE KNOWLEDGE, AND USE

Levels of Differentials in Fertility

Understanding of births (especially those that die in early infancy and mis-reporting date of birth) is important in collecting fertility data. The LDHS data indicates that the total fertility rate in Liberia is 6.5 children per woman. There is not much difference reported between rural and urban women. Women in the urban area reportedly have a total fertility rate of approximately 6.5 births. It is interesting to note that the fertility of women with some primary education is higher than those with no education and substantially higher than the fertility rate of women with secondary education. There could also be greater pregnancy wastage or under reporting of births among women with no education. A more detailed survey is necessary to detect this relationship.

Fertility Trends

Child bearing in Liberia is an activity of young women. The LDHS reports that almost 20% of teenage girls and over 25% of women 20-24 give birth in a given year. Such early child bearing has serious implications for both maternal and child health.

Completed family size in Liberia is very high. By the time a Liberian woman reaches the end of her child bearing years (usually between 45-49), she has about 7 children (6.8). Just as marriage occurs early, child bearing also occurs early, with teenage girls reporting an average of 0.5 births. The average number of live births increases with the woman's age. The distribution of women by number of births revealed that almost 40% of teenagers and 80% of women 20-24 have at least one child (Liberia and Demographic Health Survey, 1986). The proportion of mothers who become mothers in their teenage years is a basic indicator of maternal and child health. That over half of the Liberian women become mothers before they reach age 20, has serious health implications, since young mothers suffer more health problems than older mothers, and their children have higher mortality rates.

Liberia can be classified as a pronatalist culture. While women with six or more children can talk about contraceptives, it is not uncommon for them to want another child. The desire for more children usually depends on the number of children alive. According to the LDHS, 40% of the women interviewed were in need of family planning. That is they are fecund and not using contraception, despite the fact that they do not want another child in the near future. Furthermore, 22% of married women interviewed said that they intend to use contraception. in other words, not only is there a substantial need for family planning services in Liberia but also many women intended to used them.

Reproductive Health Among Adolescents, Abortion Laws, and Policies

Sexual activity among unmarried adolescents in Liberia, especially those of the urban areas has resulted in large numbers of unwanted pregnancies and illegal abortions which poses serious health and social problems. Abortion is illegal in Liberia except in cases of birth defects, threat to the mother's life, or pregnancy as result of rape. This does not stop most adolescents from seeking abortion at all cost.

The existing government and privately supported family planning programs are limited in Liberia and are targeted mostly to married couples. the use of modern contraceptive methods is very low and again limited to couples in urban areas. Virtually no data exist on the practice of family planning by adolescents (Nichols et al., 1987).

There are a number of factors that may explain the large number of pregnancies among unmarried adolescents. Besides early sexual maturity as well as marriage, the traditional social or societal norms in rural Liberia that discouraged premarital sexual activity among adolescents have been weakened by widespread urban migration.

As discussed earlier in this paper, for adolescent girls the consequences of a premarital pregnancy are serious. Besides medical complications, there are important social, education, and economic consequences. Most secondary schools in Liberia do not allow pregnant adolescents to continue their studies. The decision to terminate a pregnancy is thus necessary for those who wish to continue their education.

Substantial unmet needs exist on the part of adolescents in liberia for information concerning sexuality, reproductive health and family planning and for the provision of contraceptives services to those who are sexually active. Abortion is too high a cost for pregnant students to stay in school. Prevention strategies including the postponement of sexual activity and probably the current use of Norplant will help reduce teenage pregnancies. For those who carry their pregnancy to term, the unmarried teenage mother has limited activity, education, opportunity for upward socioeconomic mobility; a difficult future for both the mother and her child.

Traditional Practices and Customs Affecting Women's Health in Liberia

The position of the Liberian woman can be attributed to the period of colonialism or confusion brought to the Liberian society by freed slaves and the indigenous Liberian societal patterns. Some of these include female circumcision and infibulation.

Liberia is one of the oldest West African countries where female genital mutilation occurs. It is usually performed by older village women on young girls. The operation is rarely performed by skilled individuals, with surgical tools, anatomical knowledge and the use of anesthesia. Various reasons are given for the operation: preparing girls for marriage; to ensure premarital purity; lessens sexual desire and the temptation for girls and women to have intercourse before marriage. The health implications include physical and mental health consequences for women, infections, hemorrhage, and other long-term complications such as scarring of the vagina.

The extent to which female circumcision is practiced among various ethnic groups in Liberia is not known. Many women are reluctant to discuss it. I am not aware of any movement to halt this practice in Liberia and it is an uncomfortable issue to discuss since it is embedded in the culture. Any attempt to speak out against it could be seen as a gross disrespect to the elders in the society. This may explain why government officials and policy makers are reluctant to comment or take action on this issue.

Contraceptive Knowledge and Use Among Adult Women

Several studies around the world have indicated that the knowledge of contraceptives is related to its use. However, availability and accessibility of methods to couples at affordable prices are major factors in using contraceptives.

The LDHS results of 1986 indicated that 72% of the Liberians knew at least one contraceptive method. They were more likely to report having heard about modern methods (70.0%) than traditional methods (30%). The pill is the most widely used method (64%). Considering other methods, more than 40% have heard about injection and female sterilization, while around 30% were familiar with the IUDs and condoms. The percentages knowing about rhythm and withdrawal were the same—16% compared to 13% recognizing folk methods and 12% knowing about vaginal methods. Only 6% reported hearing about male sterilization. Knowledge of all methods except female sterilization were slightly lower among married women than among all women.

The LDHS also found that less than half of all respondents were familiar with a source for information about modern methods of contraception control. Age and number of children were related to knowledge, with knowledge levels highest in the 20-34 age groups. Urban women were more likely than rural women to know about a method and source of information. Educational status differentials in contraceptive knowledge were substantial. For example, 60% of currently married women who had never attended school knew modern methods as compared to 85% of those with some primary education and 95% of those with some secondary education. The religion a woman practices was also associated with the level of contraceptive knowledge and use. Knowledge of modern methods was greatest among Christian women and least among Muslim women. What does all this mean? It means that if women are to adopt family planning, they must not only know about methods but they must also be aware of a source from which they can obtain contraceptive information and services.

Approval for Use of Family Planning Methods

Among respondents to the LDHS, 28% were classified as exposed non-users. Women falling in this category were not using contraception and were having sexual intercourse. One out of four of these women cited factors related to non-use as availability, high cost, or difficulty in obtaining methods. Another fourth of the respondents feared side effects or lack of information about methods as the primary reasons they did not use contraceptives. An additional 13% said they or their husbands disapproved of the use of contraceptive methods.

The role of the Liberian male in contraceptive use cannot be ignored. Liberia is a male dominant society where males should be involved in the family planning process. It surely takes two to make a child. As most decisions in Liberian households are decided by men it is only fair to involve the men in family planning programs. Empowering women will help create the environment whereby women will want to use family planning methods even if the male partner does not agree.

In the LDHS 1986, married women were asked whether they thought their husbands approved of the use of family planning methods. Looking at the husband's perceived attitude, the results indicated that 29% of women felt that their husbands approve family planning methods, while 36% believed that their husbands disapproved of the use of contraceptives. The men were not interviewed regarding their perception of the use of contraceptives. The purpose of involving males in family planning programs is to improve communication between couples. The LDHS reported communication barriers between husbands and wives on the issue of contraceptives. Age is a factor in communication as the youngest and oldest age groups are the to not talk about family planning. As stated earlier other factors influencing communication are the education status of women, women's role in society, and the dominance of the male in the decision making process.

Prostitution and Extent of Commercial Sex

Conclusive data or information on commercial sex workers is not available. What is written here is based on personal observations and conversation with other Liberians.

There is no doubt that prostitution exists in Liberia. The extend is not known. Liberia, like many other African countries is developing rapidly. In the 1970s and 1980s there was an influx of foreign nationals to the country. Liberia also has several seaports and serves as a base for many countries, including the U.S.A. Many young people leave the small towns for big cities in search of jobs. However, many lack skills and the scarcity of jobs leaves many women stranded in cities. They resort to selling their bodies for money to live. Prostitution, however, is not widely spread. The government in the late 1970s and 1980s issued a ban on girls found soliciting men on a popular street called "Gurley Street." This did not solve the problem. The underlying factors, formed a popular location where they went to be picked up by men. The values and morals of the traditional Liberian society should be reinforced.

VIOLENCE AGAINST WOMEN

Violence against women is one of the public health issues that needs to be addressed around the world. This includes but is not limited to wife battering, rape, sexual harassment, incest, and homicide in some families. Liberia is no exception when it comes to violence against women. The extent to which these problems exist is not known as there are no data on violence against women in the Liberian society. This has not been regarded as an issue yet. Even if violence against women begins to gain ground as an issue, it is unclear how much realistic data could be collected. The claim of insufficient evidence along with social and legal barriers will serve as obstacles to acquiring accurate data on domestic violence against women.

From experience, there have been few cases of rape brought to a local hospital where I worked as an emergency room nurse. The cases seen were usually an instance where a teenage girl had been molested by an adult male. Rape is an uncomfortable topic for most physicians and nurses. Many physicians had difficulty confirming a case even with the results of clinical examination and laboratory reports. Adult cases of rape were rarely seen or discussed. This does not mean that rape does not exist. In many instances rape occurs during a date. And if a girl reports sex without her consent, she was usually told by others that she had no reason to visit a man's house if she did not want that man. However, the cases of street rape seen in countries like the U.S.A. is not common in Liberia. As a matter of fact, if a man is seen attacking a woman in the street, whether to steal from her or to rape her, others will come to her assistance immediately. This does not mean that women are not harassed in the streets.

Many wives are subject to physical abuse by their husbands. Again there are no statistics on this topic, but it is not uncommon for a woman to be brought to the emergency room at night after a beating by her husband. As in many Western countries, there are no battered women shelters. However, when a woman has been physically abused by her husband and can tolerate it no more, she can seek refuge with her parents or some relatives.

Traditionally, men are told not to beat their wives. In practice, there is a parable that most parents will used while dowering their daughter out to a man. The parents of the woman will usually tell the man,

Here is my daughter I am giving you. She has no scratches or marks on her. If for any reason you are not happy or satisfied with her behavior let me know or bring her back to me whole as she is. Do not lay your hands on her. If you put your hand on her, you have done the same to me.

At times this tradition works and in other instances it does not.

The extent to which incest occurs in the Liberian society is not known. It may not be widespread. Traditionally, there are some strict rules set for children growing up in the village. As stated earlier, in most villages or towns, parents must approve any relationship between their daughters or sons. Even if a male is considered a distant relative the girl will be prohibited from marrying that man.

There are no laws that protect women specifically against violence. Usually when a situation gets out of control, a woman has the choice of moving to her parents' compound until the crisis is resolved. More needs to be done and it is a challenge to policy makers and women's group to develop a women's health agenda in Liberia.

PARTICIPATION OF WOMEN IN PUBLIC LIFE AND LEADERSHIP

Women in Liberia have the right to vote. They make up about half of the electorate and more work in the public sector now than before. For example, in the 1980s more women were appointed to cabinet positions in government. Over the years, some of the top government positions held by women included Ministers of Health, Planning and Economic Affairs, Industry and Transportation, and Agriculture. During the 1985 elections there were a few women elected as senators and representatives for their counties. However, there are still great disparities between men and women in public life and leadership. There are no data available to confirm political participation by women.

Several prominent Liberian women have worked in the area of education. An example of positions occupied include Assistant Minister of Education. In the early 1980s the President of the University of Liberia was a female. Under her rule, the university saw many changes including good leadership and improvement in the educational standard of the university. However, men still claim a strong hold on such key positions as defense, economic policy and political affairs.

It is fair to state that unlike in some other Sub-Saharan African countries, women have always been involved in government and policy making. Women have not only held positions locally but on the international level as well. Some of these positions include ambassadors to other countries, ambassador to the

United Nations, and positions in the World Bank. Women's representation and influence in decision making is not negligible. Some of the participation is due to the so-called tie between the United States and the influence of freed slaves who returned to Liberia. If the current trend for equal opportunity continues, women will gain in education and the gap between men and women can narrow.

HEALTH IMPLICATIONS OF THE CIVIL WAR IN LIBERIA

The health status of women in Liberia is further compromised by the current civil war and its implications for the general population. The Liberian Civil War has been a tragedy. It has fanned ethnic hatred and uprooted half of the population. It has left tens of thousands dead, injured, or orphaned. There are no Liberians who can claim they are unaffected by the civil war. It has affected people of all ethnic groups, ages, and worse of all women, children and the poor. The country has a bankrupt economy with schools, hospitals and other infrastructures destroyed by the various factions in conflict. The U.S. Committee for Refugees in 1992 published an excellent document about the civil war in Liberia, *Uprooted Liberians: Casualties of a Brutal War.* Anyone interested in the Liberian crisis should read this document. The purpose of my comments here is to discuss the health impact of the civil war, especially on women and children.

The civil war has been devastating to the people of Liberia. The death toll has been high as evidenced by mass graves and by skeletons in the streets of Monrovia and its environs. Prior to the civil war, the Liberian population was 2.3 million people. The population has probably been reduced to a million by now. Is the death toll in Liberia close to 100,000? One shall never know the exact number. However, civilians in Liberia have become the target of the Liberian civil war.

The impact of war on health must be measured in a broader context as it is usually not direct fighting that claims so many lives. There is negative public health impact that induced by war. Countries torn by civil war ranked high in health indicators such as infant mortality rate, maternal mortality rate, and child mortality rates.

The war in Liberia has impacted on the health system in a variety of other ways. There has been outright destruction of physical facilities. The normal health service delivery system is broken down, forcing doctors, nurses, and other health professionals into neighboring countries in search of peace and employment. Scores of hospitals, health centers, and clinics have been abandoned, destroyed, or looted, rendering even the physical facilities useless. In Monrovia, for example, preventive public health services such as immunization and provision of potable drinking water are difficult to provide, leaving huge populations susceptible to controllable infectious diseases and epidemics. In greater Liberia, there is a decline in agriculture, transport services, commerce, and a shortage of food and money which has diminished the nutritional status of the people.

Doctors, nurses, and other medical professionals in Liberia are trained primarily in the Western tradition with the advantage that their skills are universally relevant. The disadvantage is that their training makes them readily employable in neighboring countries or in the industrialized world. The brain drain is a problem in normal times and is greatly accelerated in times of civil war or insecurity.

Civilians suffer most during any civil war. The Liberian Civil War has placed extraordinary stress on the civilian population, with women and children being the most vulnerable groups. There are pictures of 9 or 10-year-old children carrying AK-47 automatic guns bandaged by a chain of bullets. There are also reports of children being drugged and given weapons by rebel leaders to fight at the battle front. Thousands of children are homeless. Their parents have been killed in the war, in many instances in the presence of that child. There are unconfirmed reports of women tortured by gun men. At times they were raped, and then killed. There are frightening reports of pregnant women having their abdomen split open with a baronet by gun men. Several older people have been tortured and killed.

The best documented results of war are the plight of refugees. According to the United Nations High Commission on Refugees (UNHCR), there are more than 663,000 Liberian refugees in neighboring countries and more than 500,000 people displaced inside Liberia. Health and sanitary conditions in many of the refugee centers are deplorable. Malnutrition is rampant. Reaching the displaced with medical assistance is as difficult as providing for the refugees who are usually situated in one place. Just as civilians have become targets in the Liberian Civil War, so too have the public health facilities and provision of health services.

As public health services decline, medical problems increase. As insecurity mounts, fewer doctors, nurses, and paramedics are available from the normal health care delivery system. Medical supplies are quickly exhausted and shortages occur constantly. Simultaneously, the medical needs of the population increase. When emergency teams from the UN, Red Cross, and UNICEF enter these areas, they all too often concentrate on the dramatic lifesaving interventions which are usually hospital based. There is lag time between the establishment of hospital-based services and public health interventions such as immunizations and the restoration of potable water supplies. Once some peace has been achieved in Liberia between the various warring factions, it will be a great challenge for any elected government to restore optimal health to all the people of Liberia. Absolutely, the WHO goal of health for all by the year 2000 is already a failure in Liberia.

CONCLUSION

Several issues were discussed in this manuscript. Two vulnerable groups—women and children—are easily affected by diseases, social ills, economic difficulties and political oppression.

All over the world, there is a growing advocacy for women's interest. The changes being made are seen in the developed and developing countries. Despite the changes made there are still huge disparities between men and women in many Sub-Saharan countries. It fair to say that women in Liberia have enjoyed some moderate equity with men. For example, women have been able to vote and exercise their political franchise. They have also been elected to public offices and have held key positions in the government. The so-called equality is far from being met. In many instances women are still treated as second class citizens.

There are several factors that have influenced the current position of women in Liberia today. Firstly, there are deep rooted indigenous societal patterns that tend to oppress the woman in this culture. Secondly, the Liberian society has been plagued with all forms of Western ideologies that have led to total confusion of the Liberian people. Some of these ideologies were brought to Liberia by the freed slaves from America. Others were brought by Europeans trading along the west coast of Africa. Yet, a group that brought with them the "Holy Bible" also brought with them confusions which still affect the Liberian society today.

A third factor that has influenced women's position in Liberia today is the apparent lack of leadership among the women. This statement should not be misconstrued. There are several women's organizations in Liberia that have very strong leadership with clearly stated goals. But many of the women's organizations still have to get permission from the men before organizing. In the government, the President's wife (Liberia's first lady) along with the wives of other ministers of government are usually engaged in some community development activities. However, from experience, many of these organizational activities are meant to promote the political objective of their husbands. There is a need for the women of Liberia to become mobilized and self-sufficient and develop more grassroots participation.

I attempted to look at the issues that affect women's health and development in Liberia. I have written from the male perspective. This male view of women's issues illustrates that policy makers in Liberia can make policies supportive of women. Further data compilation on women's health and development is needed in the area of family life, leadership, and decision-making, health and child-bearing, education, and economic life. Such data should be collected locally and fed into an international data base system.

A crucial issue discussed in this paper was the health implications of the Liberian Civil War. The health infrastructure and economy have been destroyed by three years of civil war. It is obvious that women and children are the groups most affected by this war. Many women and children have been brutally killed.

Many of them looked on while their husbands/fathers were slaughtered like animals. Many women have been raped and tortured. There are thousands of orphans and homeless children. For example, the victims of the massacre committed by General Doe's soldiers in July 1990 at St. Peter's Lutheran Church were mostly women and children.

It is not easy to be a Liberian or an African woman at this time. It should be remembered that the Liberian woman is very unique. I speak as a male who grew up on the farm and became aware of the type of person my mother was. The Liberian woman is not just a childbearer as most men expect her to be. She makes decisions and she works very hard under the hot African sun to till the hard soil to plant grains for her family. She is willing in many instances to wear ragged clothes or to go barefoot to allow her children clothes to wear. In some instances she goes hungry to feed her children.

Women's issues in Liberia should be addressed holistically. The world needs to look at the women of Liberia. Viewed from outside, internationally, the picture changes somewhat. All women have some rights that should be universal no matter where they are. Examples include the right of a woman to vote, to go to school, own properties, be elected to public offices. However, women's health should be approached with some caution. The approach used in one country must be adapted to specific situations. The cultures of the other countries and women must be respected. While Western women are a great asset for women of the developing world, it seems only appropriate that they try not to impose their cultural values on all women. In fact, if change is to occur, it is appropriate for that change to occur from within the given culture rather than from outside influences. Changes occurring from within the culture can cause less friction and conflict and be sustained for a longer duration.

RECOMMENDATIONS

The following are broad-based recommendations that could be used to address policy issues related to women's health and development in Liberia:

1. A national women's health and development plan should be developed for women in Liberia. It should be incorporated in the national Primary Health Care Program.

2. The Government of Liberia should establish a national data base system on women and collect information relevant to the health and development of women. The Liberian Government should also endorse recommendations made by the Forty-Fifth World Health Assembly on women's health and development.

3. More reliable data on maternal deaths and research should be collected to estimate the national levels of maternal mortality. Statistics based on data from national referral hospitals such as The JFK Medical center or Phebe Hospital are not suitable for this purpose. It must be noted that several women still do not

come to the clinics or hospitals to give birth. There is a need for population based studies. Data on maternal deaths can be collected as part of prospective studies on maternal and child health or in special retrospective studies.

4. The Convention on the Rights of the Child passed by the General Assembly of the United Nations in 1989 should also be applicable to women in the case of war. International agencies will then be able to reach women caught in war situations. Children and women are the most vulnerable of the population along with the grandparents during wartime.

5. There is a need for rational design of the medical and health educational system in Liberia. In this regard, a new philosophy and doctrine of the purposes and nature of university medical education is needed. Ways of adjusting the output of universities more closely and more economically in line with the needs of the Liberian society should be conceived.

6. Steps should be taken by the government to avoid a brain drain of the health manpower. First, arrangements should be made that will enable promising young health professionals to keep abreast of developments in their own fields and maintain active contacts with their peers in other countries. This is a good way to avoid intellectual staleness which results from isolation.

In order to reduce the migration of health personnel abroad, efforts should be made to establish incentives to return to Liberia by assuring a satisfactory job on completion of training. A firm advance offer of a specific job with specified terms and conditions of employment is a strategy for change. This should include special incentives like subsidized return fares and subsidized housing as well as a reduction of import taxes on automobile and other goods brought back home.

BIBLIOGRAPHY

Aidoo, A. A. (1992). The African woman today. *Dissent, 39,* 319-325.
Airhihenbuwa, C. O. (1989). Perspectives on AIDS in Africa: Strategy for prevention and control. *AIDS Education and Prevention, 1*(1), 57-69.
Alubo, S. O. (1990). Debt crisis, health and health services in Africa. *Social Science and Medicine, 31,* 639-648.
Armijohussein, N. A. (1991). The effect of the Gulf Crisis on the children of Iraq. *New England Journal of Medicine, 235,* 977-980.
Belleh, M. (1988, December). *The Ministry of Health and Social Welfare Annual Report.* Monrovia, Liberia.
Bledsoe, C. H. (1980). *Women and marriage in Kpelle society.* Stanford, CA: Stanford University Press.
Boerma, T. (1987). The magnitude of the maternal mortality problem in Sub-Saharan Africa. *Social Science and Medicine (24),* 551-558.
Carrin, G. (1987). Community financing of drugs in Sub-Saharan Africa. *International Journal of Health Planning, 2,* 125-145.

Draper, W. H, III. (1992). Foreword. *Human development report, 1992*. New York: United Nations [Oxford University Press].

Fiedler, J. L. (1989) . Recurrent cost and public health delivery: The other war in El Salvador. *Social Science and Medicine, 25*, 876-874.

Grant, J. P. (1990). *The State of the World's Children*.. New York: UNICEF.

Johnson, D. C., Cross, A. R., Way, A. A., & Sullivan, J. M. (1988). *Demographic and health survey of Liberia*. Monrovia, Liberia: Bureau of Statistics, Ministry of Planning and Economic Affairs.

May, J. M., & McLellan, D. L. (1970). *The ecology of malnutrition in Eastern Africa and four countries of Western Africa: Equatorial Guinea, the Gambia, Liberia, Sierra Leone, Malawi, Rhodesia, Zambia, Kenya, Tanzania, Uganda, Ethiopia, the French Territory of the Afars and Issas, the Somali Republic, and Sudan*. New York: Hafner Publishing Company.

Meade, M. S. (1988). *Medical Geography*. New York: The Guilford Press.

Moran, M. H. (1990). *Civilized women: Gender and prestige in southeastern Liberia*. Ithaca, NY: Cornell University Press.

National Population Commission of Liberia. (1987). *News Letter, 1*(1).

Nichols, D., Woods, E. T., Gates, D. S., & Sherman, J. al., (1987). Sexual behavior, contraceptive practice, and reproductive health among Liberian adolescents. *Studies in Family Planning*. 18(3): 169-176.

Ojo, K. O. (1990). International migration of health manpower in Sub-Saharan Africa. *Social Science and Medicine, 31*, 631-637.

Ministry of Planning and Economic Affairs. (1987). *Population and Housing Census of Liberia-1984. Summary Results*. Monrovia, Liberia: Author.

Pragma Corporation, The. (1988, December). *Liberia, Health Sector Assessment*. Forest Church, VA: The Pragma Corporation.

Rios, R. de los, & Gomez, E. (1991, November). *Women in health and development: An alternative approach*. Paper delivered at the Fifth International Forum Association for Women in Development, Washington, DC.

Ruiz, H. A. (1992). *Uprooted Liberians: Casualties of a brutal war*. Washington, DC: U.S. Committee for Refugees.

Seager, J., & Olson, A. (1986). *Women in the world: An international atlas*. New York: Simon and Schuster.

United Nations. (1991). *The world's women 1970-1990: Trends and statistics*. (Social Statistics Indicators, series K, No. 8). New York : United Nations Publications.

Uyanga, J. (1990). Economic development strategies: Maternal and child health. *Social Science and Medicine, 31*, 649-659.

Waddington, C., & Thomas, M. (1988). Recurrent costs in the health sector of developing countries. *International Journal of Health Planning and Management, 3*, 151-166.

World Bank. (1988). Financing health services in developing countries: An agenda for reform. *PAHO Bulletin, 22*, 416-429.

3

Women's Health Status in Nigeria

Associated with The University of Illinois at Chicago WHO Collaborating Centre

Gwen Brumbaugh Keeney

SYNOPSIS OF COUNTRY

Nigeria is 356,700 square miles bordered by the Gulf of Guinea, Benin, Niger, Chad, and Cameroon (Holly, 1991). Nigeria has diverse terrains. The northern areas of Nigeria include semi-desert, savannah, and woodlands while the southern areas include swamps and tropical forests (Bair, 1991). Nigeria's natural resources include petroleum, coal, iron ore, tin, lead, zinc, columbite, and limestone. The major agricultural products in Nigeria include corn, millet, sorghum, rice, cassava, yams, cocoa, groundnuts, palm oil, and cotton. Nigeria's industries produce textiles, rubber, food products, beer, metal products, cement, lumber, car assembly, footwear, and detergent (Holly, 1991).

Nigeria has the largest population of the African countries. Recent population statistics differ considerably depending on the source.[1] The World Bank (1992) estimated a total 1990 population of 115.5 million compared to the Nigerian

---

[1]For consistency and comparisons, statistics throughout the Nigerian country profile will be based on international organizations' data rather than Nigerian census data.

government's 1991 national census report of 88.5 million. Currently, Nigeria is divided into 30 states plus the capital city of Abuja. Abuja was planned and developed as a centrally located, federal territory.

The government of Nigeria is in transition. A military government has been in power since a 1983 coup overthrew an elected government. The 1979 constitution was amended in 1984 and continued to provide legal guidance for the country (Holly, 1991). A three year plan to return to democratic elections has been implemented. Local officials were elected and installed during the first year. State officials were elected and installed during the second year. National elections were scheduled for 1992; however, the military government has postponed the final phase.

The legal system includes a dualistic governance by statutes and customary law. Both systems have their own judicial processes and court systems. The statutory legal system is based on the Constitution and is maintained by elected, military, and appointed officials. The military government has utilized military tribunals alongside the constitutional judicial system (Holly, 1991). The customary legal system incorporates the traditional ruling system of emirs, sheiks, and village chiefs. The traditional leaders operate their own court system and have compelling influence on the activities of their communities.

The government of Nigeria has ratified the Convention on the Elimination of All Forms of Discrimination against Women which became an international treaty in 1981 through the General Assembly of the United Nations (United Nations, 1991). A Directorate of Women's Affairs was established in 1987 with direct reporting to the Nigerian President. The Directorate was formed to facilitate the development and implementation of policies related to national women's programs (Akande, 1992).

DEMOGRAPHICS

Nigeria consists of 250 ethnic groups. The three largest ethnic groups are the Hausa (21%), Ibo (17%), and Yoruba (20%). Hausa, Ibo, Yoruba and English are the official languages of Nigeria (Bair, 1991; Morgan, 1984). While this report addresses a general overview of women's health issues in Nigeria, the reader is cautioned to remember that customs, traditions, and health beliefs and practices vary across ethnic groups. Thus, the content should not be generalized to the entire Nigerian population.

A large portion of the population in the north is Islamic. The people in the southern areas are more likely to be Christian. Nigeria's population is 47% Muslim, with 34% Christian, and traditional religions influence the beliefs and practices throughout Nigeria (Morgan, 1984).

Approximately 51% of the population is female, 19% of whom live in urban areas. In the urban areas the female to male ratio is 93/100 compared to the rural ratio of 105/100. The urban areas have experienced an annual total population increase of 6.1% compared to rural annual increases of 2.2% from 1985 to 1990 (AbouZahr & Royston, 1991; United Nations, 1991).

The birth rate has dropped from 1970-1980 reports of 50 to a 1990 report of 43.[2] The death rate has shown ongoing improvement from 23 in 1965 to 18 in 1975-1980 to 14 by 1990. The 1975-1980 infant mortality rate for females was 144 compared to 170 for males.[3] The 1990 total infant mortality rate has decreased to 98. Under age 5 mortality rates in 1990 were 152 for girls and 171 for boys. Forty-eight percent of females are under age 15. Forty-five percent of females are of childbearing age. The national maternal mortality rate has decreased from 1500 in 1980 to 800 by 1988.[4] Life expectancy has increased from 49 (1975-1980) to 54 years (1990) for females and from 46 to 49 years, respectively, for males. Overall life expectancy is 52 years. From 1970 to 1990, the percentage of women aged 60 and over has remained stable at 4% with a constant ratio of nearly 120 older women per 100 older men (AbouZahr & Royston, 1991; Morgan, 1984; United Nations, 1991; World Bank, 1992).

HEALTH CARE SYSTEM AND FINANCING

The Federal Ministry of Health has developed a national health care policy utilizing primary health care as the major underlying principle:

Primary health care is essential health care based on practical, scientifically sound· and socially acceptable methods and technology made universally accessible to individuals and families in the community and through their full participation and at a cost that the community and country can afford to maintain at every stage of their development in the spirit of self-reliance and self-determination. It forms an integral part both of the country's health system, of which it is the central function and main focus, and of the overall social and economic development of the community. It is the first level of contact of individuals, the family and community with the national health system bringing health care as close as possible to where people live and work, and constitutes the first element of a continuing health care process (Federal Ministry, 1988, 7-8).

---

[2]Birth and death rates are reported per 1000 total population.

[3]Infant and under age 5 mortality rates are reported per 1000 live births. Infant mortality rates may be skewed by ongoing omission of neonatal deaths of infants less than 10 days of age in some regions.

[4]Maternal mortality rates are reported per 100,000 live births.

Ransome-Kuti (1990), the Nigerian Minister of Health, has stated that the most important primary health care principle is community participation and that this corresponds with the Nigerian government's efforts to move the nation towards self-reliance, social justice, and economic reformation.

The health care system in Nigeria is structured with a Federal Minister of Health and the State Commissioners for Health functioning as a National Council on Health to oversee national guideline development and implementation. The Federal Ministry of Health provides administrative and technical support to the National Council on Health. The State Ministries of Health are comprised of State Health Advisory Committees, responsible for state planning and review of local government health budgets, and the State Hospital Management Boards which provide supervision and coordination of state hospitals and referral units. The Local Government Health Committees are responsible for delivering comprehensive health care services and collecting data in their communities. In addition, the local committees are expected to facilitate community participation and self-reliance. The committees at all levels are required to have multi-department, organization, and profession representatives from health care agencies. At the local level, the committee is required to include community leaders (Federal Ministry, 1988).

Historically, many health care services were owned and operated by religious groups and non-governmental organizations (NGOs). During the 1970s, when the Nigerian economy was strong, the Federal Government assumed ownership and management of the majority of externally owned facilities. During the 1980s, the government has encouraged some degree of return to NGO management in local areas and NGO participation on the state and local committees.

The Nigerian Constitution identifies health care as a concurrent responsibility of the national, state, and local governments. Under the national health policy, primary health care strategies are the responsibility of the local governments with support from the State Ministries of Health and guidance from the national level. Collaboration and training with traditional healers is encouraged at the local level. Secondary health care is to be provided at District and Zonal levels of the States in community hospitals or out-patient centers. Secondary care includes treating patients referred from primary care programs and providing administrative support for peripheral health care units. Tertiary care is provided at university and specialist hospitals (Federal Ministry, 1988). The majority of health care services are provided by government facilities. While most nurses and physicians are employees of the Ministry of Health, private practices and clinics can be found in urban areas and are encouraged by the national health policy.

During the 1980s, the ratio of physicians and nurses per population was 1/6410 and 1/900, respectively (World Bank, 1992). Physicians are commonly found in urban hospital settings with ratios up to 1/500 population. In rural settings the ratio is as high as 1/200,000. Nurses often staff the rural health centers; however, nurses are also found in larger numbers around urban areas.

Most of the rural health work is the responsibility of community health extension workers (Ransome-Kuti, 1990).

In addition to diagnosing and treating common conditions with simple measures, identifying pregnant women and ensuring that they deliver safely, identifying malnourished children, and providing health education in the community, the community health extension workers will mobilize the community for preventive action such as the building of latrines, wells, and roads (Ransome-Kuti, 1990, p. 205).

The national health care system includes a variety of funding sources. The Federal and State Ministries of Health provide subsidized preventive services but expect the majority of Nigerians to pay for their curative services. Nigerian households spend approximately 3% of their household income on medical expenses (World Bank, 1992). In addition, employers are encouraged to assist with the health care costs of their employees. Health insurance plans are being explored but are not widely utilized. Local communities are expected to participate in addressing financial needs of their local health care services through direct funding or through the provision of labor and materials as needed (Federal Ministry, 1988).

Previous Nigerian Ministry of Health employees stated that Nigeria spent almost 5% of the GNP on health care in 1991, which is close to the WHO recommendation of 5%. Figures from 1986 indicate that only 3% of the national health expenditure was used for primary health care programs (AbouZahr & Royston, 1991). Reports from physicians and nurses working in government facilities indicate that less money has been spent on curative services during the last few years. Decreasing curative expenditures have been associated with the Nigerian economy, increased emphasis on preventive services, and policies requiring facilities to become more self-supporting. In addition, local communities have been responsible for planning, implementing and attaining local financial resources. Utilization of local resources is difficult to document and incorporate into national expenditure statistics. Since 1986, 52 local governments were given $2,200[5] to investigate local health problems and the condition of local health resources. After follow-up workshops, the local governments were given $110,000 to implement and manage health programs developed in response to their local needs. Considerable United Nations and foreign government assistance has been provided to assist with implementing primary health care strategies in Nigeria (Ransome-Kuti, 1990).

As regards environmental health and sanitation, Nigeria has a national policy of compulsory community and household cleaning of drains, sewers, and garbage the last Saturday of each month. While enforcement is negligible, several Nigerians reported that participation was regularly observed in southern and

---

[5]Monetary values reported in dollars ($) refer to United States dollars.

western areas of Nigeria. In addition, there is a national ban on smoking in public areas.

HEALTH SERVICE UTILIZATION

Utilization of Ministry of Health facilities is affected by several factors. Staff shortages in rural areas are common. Community health aides often tend to the health care needs of their communities without additional training, supervision or local referral system. Transportation and access to equipment also limit the provision of services by health care professionals (Ofere, 1991).

Traditional health care practitioners are the predominant providers of health care services. Several different people reported that 70% of Nigerians seek assistance from traditional healers before seeking care from the scientifically trained health care workers. Traditional practitioners are able to provide accessible, affordable and culturally acceptable services. National estimates indicate that almost 80% of births are attended by traditional birth attendants (Ransome-Kuti, 1990). Regional differences are notable with Kainji Lake in western Nigeria reporting a 3% institutional birth rate compared to 79% in urban Lagos. One report indicated that the number of hospital births has decreased in conjunction with the decline in the Nigerian economy (AbouZahr & Royston, 1991). Utilization of prenatal care also varied considerably by region. Some areas in the northwest reported 8% of the women receiving prenatal care compared to some of the southern states with 80%. Interestingly, women receiving prenatal care do not necessarily give birth with a trained attendant. In the rural area of Udi, 68% of the women utilized prenatal care services with, 38% of the women having a trained attendant at the birth (AbouZahr & Royston, 1991).

Among the Yoruba in Ondo State, home remedies are generally the first response to illness. Depending on the symptoms, herbal mixtures, prayers, food changes, or baths would be used. Food patterns might be altered by withholding or providing certain foods or temperatures. Indepth discussion of traditional Yoruba healers' food proscriptions and prescriptions has been written by Odebiyi (1989). If the condition does not improve within a few days, then advice is sought from friends and family, followed by utilization of an herbalist, the local pharmacy, a clinic, or hospital. When prescribed medicines are effective, the family may decide to buy the same medicine without a prescription the next time similar symptoms occur. Local pharmacies are frequently owned and operated by merchants without any pharmaceutical training. Prescriptions are generally not required and the merchants often function as diagnosticians and prescribers. Utilization of the wrong medicine, the wrong dose, and not finishing a medicine have led to drug resistant diseases. Counterfeit drugs are not uncommon and contribute to drug interactions and more resistant diseases (Adetunji, 1991).

Utilization of health care services is often determined by families rather than individuals. Women have the basic responsibility for child care; however, important health care decisions generally require the consent of their husband or the husband's relatives. Several explanations of the need for refraining from unilateral decision making have been offered.

1. A child is not exclusively the creation of the mother and therefore components of both families need to be part of the process.
2. Men are often responsible for incurred expenses and therefore must agree to services utilized.
3. Women are expected to be deferential towards their husbands which ultimately avoids blaming and arguments (Adetunji, 1991).

A Nigerian man described the strength of his family's influence in health care decision making for his children. The husband and wife had agreed to utilize scientifically trained health care workers if their children needed health care services. His wife was caring for their two children while he was away from their home. When the children became sick, the wife consulted with her mother-in-law. The mother-in-law mandated traditional methods of facial cutting and refused to allow the children to be cared for by the local clinic. The wife felt she had no authority over her mother-in-law and complied. By the time the husband returned home, both children had died. This experience is consistent with Caldwell's (cited in Adetunji, 1991) assumption that mothers-in-law's participation in childrearing is a causative factor of high child mortality rates among illiterate mothers.

Scientifically understood causes of illness or death are not meaningful or important for many Nigerians. Underlying roots of illness and death are generally believed to be derived from curses or socially unacceptable behaviors. A Nigerian drama portrays a family's actions after the death of one of their household. The family mourned with wailing and thrashing about. Then a spiritual advisor was consulted. The cause of death was attributed to a neighboring farmer who disputed the boundary lines of their adjoining lands. The spiritualist provided something to bury in the neighbors field. When the neighbor's son was hoeing near the buried item, the son fell down and died. The skit continued the feud as revenge was sought back and forth. This understanding of disease causation has been called "remote control" by educated Nigerians as they acknowledged the tenacity of traditional beliefs even though their formal education has developed scientific understanding of disease etiologies.

NATIONAL HEALTH CONCERNS

Overall Nigerian mortality in hospitals is ascribed to infection and parasitic diseases; respiratory diseases; accidents, violence and poisoning; circulatory system diseases; and gastro-intestinal diseases (Federal Ministry, 1988). The two leading causes of death among Nigerian children under age 5 are diarrhea and respiratory infections with malaria also being a prevalent cause. Among adults the leading causes of death are road accidents, and infections, with additional mortality from chronic diseases such as diabetes, hypertension, cancer, and liver cirrhosis (Ransome-Kuti, 1990).

In Nigeria, 70,000 women die each year, which is 1 female death every 10 minutes. Twenty women have diseases per each women who dies (Baumslag, 1991b). The national maternal mortality rate was 800/100,000 births for the 1980-1990 period (United Nations, 1991). A 5-year study completed in 1981 of 22,774 hospital births in Zaria, Nigeria, reported 1045 deaths per 100,000 births (Hosken, 1988c). The difference in mortality rates could be indicative of regional differences, improvement over time, or issues of data collection and reporting. Reviews of individual hospital statistics indicate that prevailing causes of female deaths are associated with pregnancy. The causes of death include abortion, puerperal sepsis, uterine hemorrhages, hypertension (toxemia), ectopic pregnancies, and obstructed labors with associated uterine rupture or prolapse. In addition, maternal deaths can be associated with social and cultural influences on Nigerian women. It has been common for women to begin childbearing at early ages, with closely spaced pregnancies until their death or onset of menopause. Inadequate or poor delivery of health care services such as intrauterine device (IUD) insertions, abortions, manual removal of placentas, and development of antibiotic resistance have also increased maternal mortality (Harrison, 1988; Ofere, 1991).

Another common practice has been for women to eat after the men have completed their meal. Among poor families, the combination of pregnancies and limited food intake results in depletion of nutritional stores and diminished ability for women to survive pregnancies and infections. Sixty-five percent of Nigerian women are anemic during pregnancy (Seager & Olson, 1986). Anemia in women is prevalent countrywide and has been identified as the main cause of 3 to 12% of hospital maternal deaths. In Kaduna State, anemia was the main cause of 46% of maternal deaths for women without prenatal care (AbouZahr & Royston, 1991). Malnutrition also contributes to high percentage of low birth weight infants. In 1979, 15 to 20% of infants had low-birth weights. Statistics from 1985 indicate that 25% of newborns had low birth weights (World Bank, 1992).

In Zaria area, 25% of childbearing women have stunted growth related to malnutrition. The frequent combination of adolescent pregnancies and stunted growth increase the potential for obstructed labors and associated complications. Nutritional supplementation and utilization of medications for malaria and intestinal parasites has been shown to increase the height of a significant proportion of women with first pregnancies and reduce the proportion of abdominal deliveries compared to untreated primiparas (AbouZahr & Royston, 1991).

Ahmadu Bello University Hospital in Kaduna State's 1988 statistics indicate a maternal mortality rate (MMR) of 2,833. When the MMR is divided according to age and prenatal care, females under age 16 without prenatal care had rates above 5,500, while women over age 16 with prenatal care had MMRs between

90 and 160. Fifteen percent of Nigerian births occur among women over age 35. The combination of increased age and parity multiply the risk of maternal death. Parity greater than 5 generally doubled the maternal mortality rates among adult women without prenatal care, yet the MMR remained near 150 if prenatal care was provided. Women with some formal education generally participated in prenatal care programs. The MMR among formally educated women was 246 compared to 1,155 among women without any formal education. Religious affiliation also was associated with differences in maternal mortality rates. Among Christian women, the MMR was 154. Women identified as Islamic had a MMR of 1,596. Women from other religious backgrounds had the lowest MMR of 118 (AbouZahr & Royston, 1991). Education, age, prenatal care and religious practices are interrelated and provide a context for appraising maternal health in Nigeria.

Vesico-vaginal fistulas (VVF) are a serious women's health concern in Nigeria. Vesico-vaginal fistulas are openings between the vagina and the bladder which cause urinary incontinence. The accompanying hygiene problems include infections, unpleasant odor, and limitation of social interactions. Recto-vaginal fistulas may occur in conjunction with VVF. The incidence is highest in areas where females marry at younger ages and begin having children before their pelvic bones have fully developed. About one-third of women with VVF are teenagers. Other causative factors of VVF are the deleterious practice of vaginal application of rock salt during labor or insertion of caustic herbal pessaries into the vagina (Harrison, 1988). In the Zaria, Nigeria area, maternal death and vesico-vaginal fistulas were absent among women who had completed secondary education compared to a maternal mortality rate of 40,000/100,000 for pregnant girls aged 15 or less in the same communities (Hosken, 1988c).

VVF is a health and social problem. Repair centers are developing as a new strategy to provide physical repair and social support for ostracized women. Women who come to VVF centers are taught economically viable skills which have been used to make salable items to sustain the centers and provide the women with an income (Baumslag, 1991b; Ojanuga, 1992).

Human Immunodeficiency Virus (HIV) statistics are not available from the Nigerian Ministry of Health for public information. Verbal reports from health professionals indicate that the incidence is quite low. The Nigerian Ministry of Health has launched a nationwide HIV prevention campaign through the mass media. Radio spots, prominently placed posters, and public discussions have been utilized. Public awareness of HIV existence is high. A study of college students found that a majority of the students knew accurate information about how HIV is contracted. Among the student group, 65% were sexually active with only 13% utilizing condoms (Okeke, 1992). The study recommended prevention strategies which incorporated religious considerations and providing additional safe sex information to women. Women face several cultural and social barriers related to self-protection from HIV. Polygamy is common, therefore married women are exposed to husbands with multiple sexual contacts. Attempts to use condoms implies mistrust of any one of the marital group's fidelity. Another social belief is that condoms are only used for promiscuous sex and therefore a woman suggesting condom use is viewed as unfaithful or as a prostitute.

Nigerian figures from 1980, indicate that 26 to 50% of the population had safe drinking water sources (Seager & Olson, 1986). An example of implementing primary health care concepts for improved water resources is a case study from Mapo Community in Ibadan, Nigeria. A research team from the University of Ibadan conducted unstructured interviews at the Mapo roundabout. Of 100 subjects, 60 were women. All 60 women identified an adequate water supply as their most pressing need. The traditional women's roles included fetching water, home sanitation, and preparation of food and beverages. In addition, women were identified as influential in shaping family attitudes, discipline, and social and health practices. Therefore the research team developed safe water educational interventions targeting house women and women food sellers. Local health center staff and health committees organized 65 women into five groups. Educational strategies included health talks, health education songs, demonstration of water purification, identification of quick learners for inclusion in the teaching process as role models/demonstrators, in-home small group practice, and open question and dialogue sessions. Post-intervention evaluation included produce market and home observations. Visible changes in cleanliness and water storage were evident and the women involved in the groups had begun lobbying the local health committee to provide protection for the wells (Olaseha & Namanja, 1985-86).

EDUCATIONAL ACHIEVEMENT FOR WOMEN

The Nigerian Minister of Education has been credited with saying, "Educate a woman, educate a nation." In general, males have had more access to formal education than females. Social norms are changing, resulting in increased numbers of females participating in formal education. It is interesting to note that some Nigerian fathers have stated that financial gain has been their motivation for educating their daughters. Educated women are able to contribute more to the income of their households; therefore, the bride price is expected to reflect the women's earning potential.

Literacy rates demonstrate the effect of increasing enrollments in formal education. The 1977 literacy rates were 6% for females and 25% for males. By 1985, literacy rates were 23% for females and 45% for males and showed continued gains in 1990 to 39% and 51%, respectively. In 1975, 32% of girls and 45% of boys (ages 6-11) were enrolled in primary school. Reports from 1986-1989 give enrollment ranges of 63-85% for girls and up to 97% for boys at the primary level. The ratio of girls to boys in primary school had improved to 82/100 by 1989. At the secondary level (ages 12-17), 14% of the girls and

24% of boys were enrolled in 1975. Reports from 1989 do not reveal much improvement at the secondary level, with total enrollment of 19% and female enrollment at 16%. The 1989 secondary school ratio of females to males was 75/100. The ratio of 20-24 year old Nigerian women to men in post-secondary school was less than 30/100 in 1985. The overall enrollment in post-secondary school for 1989 was only 3% (AbouZahr & Royston, 1991; Morgan, 1984; Seager & Olson, 1986; United Nations, 1991; World Bank, 1992).

As with health care services, teacher availability has been limited. The national ratio of primary school students per teacher was reported at 37 (World Bank, 1992). School buildings and teachers are sparsely distributed in many rural areas resulting in larger student/teacher ratios than in urban areas. The Nigerian government has subsidized post-secondary education for men and women in Nigeria and abroad. Current government practice encourages Nigerian students to attend Nigerian universities when their desired course of study is available. Women have entered professional degree programs facilitating their entry into law, medicine, education, government, media, and business (Hosken, 1988a).

The University of Ibadan has established a Women's Research and Documentation Centre (WORDOC) within their Institute of African Studies. WORDOC provides a base for promoting, funding, collecting, and disseminating research related to multi-disciplinary women's issues in Nigeria. WORDOC has actively participated in networking with international women's research groups (Hosken, 1989b).

ECONOMICS

A decline in the Nigerian economy can be identified by contrasting the May 1983 Nigerian Naira value of 1/$1.45 (Morgan, 1984) to the November 1992 Naira value of 1/$24. Another example of the changing economic status is the Gross National Product (GNP) per capita in 1980 of $1010 (Morgan, 1984) compared to the 1990 GNP per capita of $290 (World Bank, 1992). If the 1991 Nigerian census population report is utilized, then the GNP per capita would need to be adjusted upward to approximately $380. A measure of the severity of economic distress is the increasing external debt. The 1975 external debt was $1.14 billion which had increased to $30.72 billion by 1988 (International Economics, 1990). While many factors affect the Nigerian economy, the fluctuation in petroleum revenues has had considerable impact on national development and decline. Nigeria received $700 million in 1970 with an increase to $25 billion in 1980 for petroleum. By 1986, oil income had dropped to $6 billion with some improvement in 1991 to $13 billion. National discussions related to economic recovery and reform indicated that Nigerians prefer self-imposed austerity measures rather than reliance on International Monetary Fund loans (Holly, 1991).

The national economic policies have encouraged development of cooperatives. Women in several parts of Nigeria have effectively utilized cooperatives for economic development and been receptive to innovations. Women's cooperatives in Ile-Ife area have operated credit programs, joint farming ventures, and collective marketing strategies (Akande, 1992). Historically, the International Institute of Tropical Agriculture in Ibadan, Nigeria, has focused on increasing crop yields and teaching the improved strategies to men in agricultural communities. When an expatriate woman redirected the teaching methods to women and included the additional topics of nutrition, food processing, and utilization, the women began communal farming (in addition to their normal work load). The results have included considerable increases in crop yields, improved storage, and increased income related to the increases in quantity and longevity (Hosken, 1988d).

"Women have always had economic power and have exerted influence in Nigerian society through women's councils or through family connections" (Hosken, 1988a, p. 6). Women living in seclusion are also reported to be economically active by utilizing emissaries to sell their products (Ogundipe-Leslie, 1984). In polygamous relationships, the women have usually needed to be financially resourceful to care for the needs of their children and themselves. Nationwide, 46% of women are economically active compared to 88% of the men. Females have comprised 35% of the total paid workforce from 1970 to the present. Statistics from 1980 to 1987 indicate that 42% of female workers are in unpaid work activities such as agricultural and household tasks. Only 9% of the total workers are unpaid. Of the total female workers, 37% were identified as employers and 18% were identified as employees (International Economics, 1990; Seager & Olson, 1986; United Nations, 1991).

Regional and ethnic differences influence women's occupational activities. For instance, an essential part of Yoruba women's lives is trading or income-generating endeavors (Akande, 1992). Nigerian women provide 40% of the agricultural labor. National statistics indicate that 39% of employed women are in sales, 23% are primary school teachers, 19% are secondary level teachers, 10% are university teachers, 12% are involved with production and crafts, 6% are in executive or administrative roles, 1.5% are professional or technical workers, and 0.5% are clerical workers (Morgan, 1984).

The government of Nigeria has supported the rights of women workers through national legislation mandating equal pay for men and women, legislating at least 12 weeks of maternity leave without mandatory pay, and by signing the International Labour Organization (ILO) convention setting standards for women's work opportunities (Seager & Olson, 1986). Nevertheless, implementation of policy is not enforced, enabling women's wages to be 66% of men's wages in some areas (Morgan, 1984).

Retired workers generally receive pensions from their employers. Traditionally, the extended family attends to the needs of their aging relatives. Nigerian adults described an unwavering sense of responsibility to care for their mothers' financial and health needs. When families were geographically separated, money would be sent or leaves from work would be arranged to attend to the needs of aging or ill parents. More recently, the government has operated a few homes for the elderly with family members required to assist with the financial costs (Morgan, 1984).

FAMILY STRUCTURE

Nigerians are generally expected to marry. Nationwide, more than 50% of Nigerian females age 15 to 19 have married (Seager & Olson, 1986). The average age of first marriage for Nigerian females is 18.7 (AbouZahr & Royston, 1991). The legal minimum age for marriage is 12 for females and 14 for males, with mutual and parental consent required until age 21 (Morgan, 1984). Islamic and Christian communities differ in the age of marriage of females. In Christian communities marriages tend to be postponed until females are in their late teens or young adults and generally have allowed couples to choose their partners. Younger marriage age is more frequent among Muslim females, and in some areas customary laws do not require consent of the bride (Seager & Olson, 1986). Extended family relationships are important factors in marriage and family decision-making. The groom's family generally provides a bride-price to the bride's family. Among some groups, the bride's family might be expected to provide a dowry to the groom.

Polygyny is a common practice, with about half of all married women in one western region living in polygamous unions (Ware, 1979). Four wives is the maximum allowed among faithful Islamic families. Polygamous household arrangements vary. Muslim husbands are supposed to provide separate dwellings for each of their wives and the children live with their birth mothers. This can be contrasted with some traditional polygamous families where the wives are helpmates for each other (the first wife may have even decided when and who the husband will marry next) with all the women and children living together as one family. Adult Nigerians have reported that they feel love and responsibility towards all the mothers from their compound and do not know or need to know which woman is their birth mother.

Ethnic and customary practices differ in relation to a woman's ownership and control of assets. Statutory law enables women to own and control assets brought into and earned during marriage. Traditionally, Yoruba men have maintained ownership of marital property while Hausa men and women have practiced joint ownership of assets. In Nigeria, Islamic teaching prohibits women from managing property or disposing of more than one-third of the marital assets unless her husband consents (Morgan, 1984). Another property issue occurs when men die without leaving a will. Because couples can marry through customary law,

Muslim law, and legislative law, the property rights of widows vary. Legislative law provides protection of assets for women and children following a man's death. However, marriages through customary law in Benue State enable the male kin of the deceased to inherit all the property including the widow (Angagende, 1992).

The fertility rate has remained near 7 births per woman from 1970 to 1990 (United Nations, 1991). Women in polygamous marriages tend to have a lower fertility rate than women in monogamous marriages (Ukaegbu, 1977). A contraception prevalence rate of only 5% was reported for the early 1980s (AbouZahr & Royston, 1991). The National Health Policy highlights family planning as part of the minimum health services to be provided nationwide. Family planning is defined as preventing unplanned pregnancies, child-spacing, limiting family size, and achieving desired pregnancies (Federal Ministry, 1988). An example of a primary health care strategy utilized to promote family planning is the Ibadan Market Project. Market traders were provided with comprehensive family planning, reproductive, and basic illness training and then supplied with contraceptives, malaria medications, and oral rehydration packets to include as commodities in their market stalls. Women traders were found to be very effective sales agents of contraceptives and illness treatments (Ladipo, Otolorin, Delano, Weiss, & McNamara, 1986).

Breastfeeding in Nigeria has followed trends in other countries. When the Nigerian economy was strong, women often returned to their education or employment within 6 weeks of birth. Artificial milk was utilized for infant feeding with the belief that this practice was safe if orange juice and water supplements were provided to prevent infant constipation. Subsequently, infant mortality increased in conjunction with the increased occurrences of infant diarrhea. The decline in the economy has influenced many women to choose breastfeeding as a cost effective feeding method and to provide a safe form of child spacing (Babalola, 1989). An informal policy in the public sector enables women to return home for an hour each day for breastfeeding or other family responsibilities (Morgan, 1984).

Divorce is not common but can be granted through the statutory or customary systems. The statutory process requires mutual consent and a 2 year separation. Without consent, statutory grounds include nonconsummation, adultery, desertion, or 3 years of separation. Statutory law enables either partner to receive alimony or child custody. Divorce through customary law can occur without any court process by the wife departing voluntarily or in response to the husband's command. Customary courts can grant a divorce by decree, which is almost exclusively the husband's privilege. Customary law generally requires the wife's family to return the bride-price to the husband and for the children to be raised by the husband or his family (Morgan, 1984). The traditional loyalty between Nigerian mothers and their children has reportedly led to husbands' requesting their wives to return and relieve the stresses experienced in relation to the children.

SEXUALITY

Nigerian women's dress reflects a variety of social influences. Brightly colored cloth with locally printed or tie-dyed patterns is used for dresses or as a skirt wrap with matching tops and head scarfs. European dress is often found in schools and work settings. Pants or trousers are rarely worn by most Nigerian women. In Kano State, Islamic women wear a loosely wrapped cloth over their dress. The cloth covers the hair and extremities without veiling the face. Seclusion of women, or purdah, is practiced in some Islamic communities in Nigeria.

The Nigerian Health Ministry has documented the practice of female circumcision in every state. The Medical Women's Association of Nigeria's research found that 90% of girls in eight states were still being circumcised with regional estimates ranging from 50% to 100%. The predominant method of female circumcision in Nigeria is excision of the clitoris. About 15% of females are circumcised by infibulation (Hosken, 1988b). In some areas, specifically the north-central region, infibulation is practiced with removal of the clitoris, labia minora, part of the labia majora, and tightly closing the vaginal opening (Seager & Olson, 1986). The Igbo, living in south-eastern Nigeria, have a 97% excision rate generally performed on 8-day-old newborns (Hosken, 1989a). In south-western Nigeria, *Olola* families are the traditional circumcisers among the Yoruba. Generally, men circumcise males and women circumcise females. Circumcision practitioners include barbers and physicians (Hosken, 1980).

While some families are not choosing to continue the practice, the beliefs related to circumcision still influence family interactions. A Nigerian doctor reported an incident of prolonged labor which the mother-in-law believed was caused by the absence of circumcision. The mother-in-law insisted that a circumcision be done during the labor to enable the birth to occur. After the physician agreed to do an excision and moved the laboring woman to another room, the labor progressed adequately without circumcision.

Female circumcision complications include hemorrhage, shock related to no anesthesia, local and systemic infections, tetanus, urinary obstruction or infections, dysmenorrhea, infertility, keloids, painful intercourse, absence of female orgasm, childbirth complications including vesico-vaginal fistulas and maternal or fetal death, and psychological effects (Hosken, 1980).

An 11-state community health education project related to harmful effects of female circumcision was begun in 1988 by the National Association of Nigerian Nurses & Midwives (Hosken, 1989a). Nigeria has sent delegations to several international conferences related to female circumcision and formed a National

Committee in 1985. The National Committee promotes the discontinuation of female circumcision by providing educational services to professionals, market women, traditional practitioners, and international organizations (Hosken, 1988b).

Abortion is illegal and a cultural taboo in Nigeria unless the woman's life is in danger. Legal requirements include a court order and two physicians' diagnoses. Stiff penalties up to 14 years in prison can be levied against women and the practitioners involved in abortion (Morgan, 1984). In spite of the strict moral and legal codes, Nigerian nurses in the northern areas reported seeing many women in their hospitals for abortion complications. The University of Benin Teaching Hospital, in southern Nigeria, admits 25% of their gynecology patients for abortion-related conditions and reported 22% of maternal deaths from 1973 to 1985 were caused by abortions (AbouZahr & Royston, 1991). A 1974 report indicated that 5/1000 women in western Nigeria died each year from illegal abortion (Morgan, 1984). In western Nigeria, private abortion services can be obtained from health care professionals. In other regions, traditional practitioners provide a large portion of abortion services.

Verifiable information related to abortion prevalence, complications, and personnel is not readily accessible because of the legal and moral prohibitions in Nigeria. Causes of maternal deaths related to illegal abortions are generally documented according to the predominant consequence. Sepsis is frequently identified as the cause of death after abortions. Sepsis accounts for 6 to 10% of maternal deaths reported by most regional Nigerian hospitals. In northern Nigeria, Plateau and Kaduna State hospitals reported sepsis as the cause of 13 to 15% of maternal deaths (AbouZahr & Royston, 1991).

Prostitution or participation in merchandized sexual activity is illegal throughout Nigeria. Historically, prostitution has been socially acceptable in some regions. Professional prostitutes reportedly have had a union and, in 1950, initiated two civil rights organizations (Morgan, 1984).

VIOLENCE AND WOMEN

Domestic violence is known to occur in all regions of Nigeria, with wives being the most frequent target of physical abuse. Health care professionals state that wife beatings are often severe and require medical intervention. Some legal aid is supposed to be available for abused women; however, police do not provide immediate assistance (United Nations, 1991). Nigerian young men acknowledge the widespread occurrence of wife beating and state that the incidence is decreasing. While laws are not changing, formally educated young adults' values related to marriage and women seem to be moving towards increased partnership between men and women. Incest and domestic homicide are reportedly rare occurrences and would have serious social consequences if publicly discovered.

Rape is considered a major social and moral taboo among Nigerians. The incidence is reported to be extremely low with less than 5 offenses per 100,000 population. At the same time, it is not a criminal offence for a husband to rape his wife (Seager & Olson, 1986). A husband can be prosecuted for assault if he uses physical force to have intercourse with his wife (Morgan, 1984).

Nigerian national crime statistics in the early 1980s indicate that 5% to 10% of all persons arrested were women (Seager & Olson, 1986). Amnesty International reported that executions were done in Nigeria during 1991; however, gender differences were not provided (cited in Utne, 1992).

WOMEN'S STRENGTHS

"The greatest strength of Nigerian women lies in their right and ability to work, in addition to their resourcefulness and great capacity for emotional survival" (Ogundipe-Leslie, 1984, p. 503).

Historically, Nigerian women have been active and effective participants in the economy and rural life. As in other parts of the world, women's contributions to the social fabric have not been adequately documented and therefore development projects have not attended to improvement of women's roles or women's participation. Even current Nigerian literature emphasizing the community development principle of inclusive community participation does not necessarily incorporate women into the process. An example is portrayed by the methodology used to assess community development processes in three regions of Nigeria. Assessment was accomplished by interviewing heads of households, and a snowball strategy used to identify and interview village leaders (Adejunmobi, 1990). No gender statistics were reported; however, women would rarely fill the roles selected for interviews.

Maryam Babangida, the First Lady of Nigeria, has been instrumental in the development of the Better Life for Rural Women Programme. The Better Life Programme was created out of an awareness of the absence of women in Nigerian development programs. Nigerians have noted that the program has been beneficial, especially in providing health education. However, Nigerians have intimated that the largest proportion of program's services have not been provided to the targeted rural women. Since the management is located in urban areas under the direction of governors' wives, urban women have greater relational and logistical access to the Better Life staff and programs.

A number of women's organizations are active and have been effective resources for Nigerian women. The National Council of Women's Organizations in Nigeria has organized educational programs for women factory workers to teach health risk reduction and relevant rights (Baumslag, 1991a). The Committee for Women in Development operates nationally with state units. The National Council of Women's Societies of Nigeria (NCWS) is a non-partisan organization comprised of individuals and women's religious, social, humanitarian, and cultural groups. NCWS provides child care, education and political action services intended to decrease women's burdens and promote women's full participation in community life (Hosken, 1986).

Nigerian women continue to attend to the maternal role described as bearers, socializers, and nurses of the subsequent generation. In addition, women's normal roles include occupational, economic, domestic, conjugal, family, individual, and community roles (Akande, 1992).

POLITICAL PARTICIPATION OF WOMEN

The 1979 Nigerian Constitution prohibits discrimination based on sex, ethnicity, religion, language, or status. In 1983, five women served as Federal government ministers, two women were members of the Senate and one woman was in the Nigerian House of Representatives (Morgan, 1984). In 1987, women comprised 4.3% of the decision-makers in the Federal ministries, without any women serving in the top positions within their ministries (United Nations, 1991). Before the national elections were postponed, two women were campaigning to be the Nigerian President.

Historically, women received the right to vote in 1954. Because of the dualistic governmental authority, women's voting privileges varied by region until 1977 when women's right to vote became a national standard (Morgan, 1984). In the southern and western regions, a larger proportion of women reportedly exercise their right to vote than men. In the northeastern part of Nigeria several Nigerians stated that some women have been prevented from voting by their husbands, while two expatriates reported seeing women well-represented in ballot lines.

Historically, many Nigerian women have played key leadership roles among their people. Amina, Queen of Zaria, ruled the Hausa people in the 15th century. During the 1800s, Yoruba women had significant political positions in the Oyo Kingdom, including royal treasurer, guardian of royal graves and influential titles as mothers of the king or crown prince. Among the Ibo, the women have been rebuilding the traditional women's social system. The traditional Ibo system included a woman as village Omu with her female cabinet and policewomen to maintain marketplace order. A regular Ibo women's meeting to discuss women's issues, called the *mikiri*, created rules related to women's economic life and identified collective strategies for managing domestic roles (Morgan, 1984).

During British rule, traditional women's systems were overlooked. Taxation of women's holdings and the usurpation of women's influential roles have been identified as major causes of the Women's War of 1929, or Aba Riots as named by British writers. Nigerian women have utilized collective action for strikes and violence, as well as derisive song and dance, to successfully thwart unacceptable forays into the women's domain (Morgan, 1984).

Nigerian men have commented that they appreciate Nigerian women because the women continue to show kindness and respect to men even as the women gain power and authority. An example has been Ladi Adamu, a local government council member in Kano State. Ladi Adamu is a mother, a Muslim, wears traditional Fulani shawls over her head and shoulders, and seeks her husband's approval of her political participation. She has promoted women's rights through traditional language and mores and has facilitated immunization, education, the building of wells, water pumps, and roads in rural areas. Attitudes are changing and Ladi Adamu received the most votes of any local candidate during the Kano State elections. Nevertheless, the Chairman of her local council advised her to marry a councillor if she wanted to influence the local council. (Hosken, 1988e).

Women are eligible to serve voluntarily in the military in non-combatant roles, primarily in the medical corps.

OTHER ASPECTS OF INTEREST TO WOMEN'S HEALTH

The Population Crisis Committee (1988) provided a summarized evaluation of five components of well-being among women in 99 countries. Nigeria ranked above three countries in women's health indicators, such as female life expectancy with gender differentials, and female mortality rates during infancy, childhood and the childbearing years. The indicators related to marriage and children included female age of marriage, fertility rates, utilization of contraceptives, and gender ratios of post-married singles. The marriage and children score for Nigeria was above five countries. In education, Nigeria scored higher than 18 countries based on female school enrollment, literacy rates, and proportion of women teachers in secondary schools. Nigeria's ranking for women and employment was higher than 28 countries based on the percentage of women employed, self-employed, and in professional roles, and the percent of females in the total work force. The fifth component was social equality of women. Nigeria scored above five countries in reference to political, legal, economic, marital, and family equality.

"Most middle-class Nigerian women will agree that the basic situation of women in Nigeria is not intolerable or appalling because of the economic opportunities women have within the system" (Ogundipe-Leslie, 1984, p. 498). Women and development programs in Nigeria have successfully improved safe water supplies, agricultural yields, and economic income. Decreased birth rates and improved maternal and infant mortality rates have occurred since the Nigerian Ministry of Health began promoting primary health care strategies. While efforts to reestablish traditional women's organizations and rekindle women's cooperative strategies have led to improvements in participants' general well-being, access to formal education and scientifically trained health care workers are major determinants in the physical health and safety of women and their children.

Note: The author extends appreciation to the many Nigerian and expatriate individuals who endured interviews and offered their thoughts and experiences. The author is from the United States, visited Nigeria in 1992 with a brief tour of health care services, and would not have written this paper without the support and assistance of women and men from Nigeria.

REFERENCES

AbouZahr, C. & Royston, E. (1991). *Maternal mortality: A global factbook.* Geneva: World Health Organization.

Adejunmobi, A. (1990). Self-help community development in selected Nigerian rural communities: Problems and prospects. *Community Development Journal, 25,* 225-235.

Adetunji, J. A. (1991). Response of parents to five killer diseases among children in a Yoruba community, Nigeria. *Social Science & Medicine, 32,* 1379-1387.

Akande, M. (1992). Enhancing the performance of women's multiple roles: A case study of Isoya Rural Development Project, Ile-Ife, Nigeria. *Community Development Journal, 27*(1), 60-68.

Angagende, C. (1992). Widowhood rites in Nigeria. *Women's International Network News, 18*(4), 55.

Babalola, M. (1989, Spring). From Nigeria: Ups and downs. *Women's International Public Health Network News, 5,* 7.

Bair, F. E. (Ed.). (1991). *Countries of the world and their leaders:Yearbook 1991.* Detroit: Gale Research Inc.

Baumslag, N. (Ed.). (1991a, Spring). International womens [*sic*] health: Manilla [*sic*], Nov. 1990. *Women's International Public Health Network News, 9,* 8.

Baumslag, N. (Ed.). (1991b, Winter). Making a difference. *Women's International Public Health Network News, 10,* 17.

Federal Ministry of Health. (1988). *The national health policy and strategy to achieve health for all Nigerians.* Lagos, Nigeria: Author.

Harrison, K. A. (1988). Maternal morbidity. *Women's International Network News, 14*(2), 22-23.

Holly, S. (Ed.). (1991). *Background notes* (Publication No. 7953). Washington, DC: United States Department of State, Bureau of Public Affairs, Office of Public Communication.

Hosken, F. P. (1980). *Female sexual mutilations: The facts and proposals for action.* Lexington, MA: Women's International Network News.

Hosken, F. (Ed.). (1986). Reports from around the world: Middle East and Africa. *Women's International Network News, 12*(1), 56-64.

Hosken, F. (Ed.). (1988a). Country reports on human rights. *Women's International Network News*, *14*(2), 4-11.

Hosken, F. (Ed.). (1988b). International seminar: Female circumcision strategies to bring about change. *Women's International Network News*, *14*(3), 24-31.

Hosken, F. (Ed.). (1988c). Maternal health in Sub-Saharan Africa. *Women's International Network News*, *14*(2), 23-24.

Hosken, F. (Ed.). (1988d). New farming methods for women in Nigeria. *Women's International Network News*, *14*(2), 47.

Hosken, F. (Ed.). (1988e). The status of women in Islamic northern Nigeria. *Women's International Network News*, *14*(4), 40.

Hosken, F. (Ed.). (1989a). Genital and sexual mutilations of females. *Women's International Network News*, *15*(1), 28-29.

Hosken, F. (Ed.). (1989b). Reports from around the world: Africa. *Women's International Network News*, *15*(1), 40-47.

International Economics Department of the World Bank. (1990). *World tables 1989-90* (Data on Diskette). Washington, D.C.: The International Bank for Reconstruction and Development/The World Bank.

Ladipo, O. A., Otolorin, E. O., Delano, G. E., Weis, E., & McNamara, R. (1986). The Ibadan market project: An urban model for delivery of community-based health and family planning services. *Planner's Forum Magazine*, *2*(1), 16-24.

Morgan, R. (1984). *Sisterhood is global*. Garden City, NY: Anchor Press.

Odebiyi, A. I. (1989). Food taboos in maternal and child health: The view of traditional healers in Ile-Ife, Nigeria. *Social Science & Medicine*, *28*, 985-996.

Ofere, C. M. (1991, Winter). Maternal morbidity and mortality, Nigeria. *Women's International Public Health Network News*, *10*, 4.

Ogundipe-Leslie, M. (1984). Nigeria: Not spinning on the axis of maleness. In R. Morgan, *Sisterhood is Global* (pp. 498-504). Garden City, NY: Anchor Press.

Ojanuga, D. (1992, November). *Birth injury in African communities: VVF among the women of Northern Nigeria*. Poster session presented at the 120th Annual Meeting of the American Public Health Association, Washington, D.C.

Okeke, M. U. (1992). *Community-based strategies for preventing HIV infection among Nigerian young adults*. Poster session presented at the 120th Annual Meeting of the American Public Health Association, Washington, D.C.

Olaseha, I. O. & Namanja, G. B. (1985-86). Focusing on women for water and sanitation: The case of Mapo Community in Ibadan, Nigeria. *International Quarterly of Community Health Education*, *6*, 335-343.

Population Crisis Committee. (1988, June). Country rankings of the status of women: Poor, powerless and pregnant. *Population Briefing Paper*, *20*.

Ransome-Kuti, O. (1990). Nigeria: Developing the primary health care system. In E. Tarimo & A. Creese (Eds.), *Achieving health for all by the year 2000: Midway reports of country experiences*. Geneva: WHO.

Seager, J. & Olson, A. (1986). *Women in the world: An international atlas*. New York: Simon & Schuster.

Ukaegbu, A. O. (1977). Fertility of women in polygynous unions in rural eastern Nigeria. *Journal of Marriage and the Family, 39*, 397-403.

United Nations. (1991). *The world's women 1970-1990: Trends and statistics* (Social Statistics and Indicators, Series K, No.8). New York: United Nations Publications.

Utne, E. (Ed.). (1992, November/December). The company we keep. *Utne Reader, 54*, p. 96.

Ware, H. (1979). Polygyny: Women's views in a transitional society, Nigeria 1975. *Journal of Marriage and the Family, 41*, 185-195.

World Bank. (1992). *World development report 1992: Development and the environment*. Oxford: Oxford University Press.

4

Women's Health Status in South Africa

Associated with The University of Illinois at Chicago WHO Collaborating Centre

Sophie Makhubu

COUNTRY AND DEMOGRAPHICS

The Republic of South Africa lies at the southern tip of the African continent. The country has a narrow coastal zone and an extensive interior plateau with altitudes ranging from 1,000 to 2,000 meters above sea level. South Africa lacks important arterial rivers or lakes, so extensive water conservation and control are necessary. The coastline is about 4,300 kilometers long. The country has a moderate climate with sunny days and cool nights. The 1990 census indicated a population of 35,282,000 and a growth rate of 2.2%. South African law divides the population into four major groups (Table 4-1). Africans descended mainly from Sotho and Nguni people; Whites from Dutch, French, English, and German settlers, with small admixtures of other European people. Whites speak Afrikaans or English, both official languages. Coloreds are mostly descendants of indigenous peoples and the earliest European and Malays settlers, and Asians are mainly descendants of Indian workers brought to South Africa in the mid-19th century to work as indentured laborers on sugar estates in Natal. In South Africa there is an apartheid form of government. Although many legal aspects of apartheid are being dismantled, significant legal inequalities remain and the social effects of years of inequality persist.

Table 4-1. Population by Race

Category	Total Number	Percentage
Africans	25,403,040	72
Whites	5,645,120	16
Coloreds	3,175,380	9
Asians	1,058,460	3

Source: Demographic Yearbook, 1990.

Health Concerns and Health Demographics

South Africa's rapid population growth has resulted in the expansion of the South African population from 5 million at the beginning of this century to well over 30 million in the 1980s. A further doubling of the population is projected over the next 25-30 years. Simultaneously there has been rapid influx into urban areas with resulting growth of peri-urban settlements for which totally inadequate health care facilities have been created. Aging of the population, poverty, and disruption of the family pose additional medico-social challenges to the delivery of health care. Population growth and unemployment have outstripped the development of educational and other social facilities necessary for healthy living.

South Africa exhibits distinctive features of both developed and less developed countries; Whites have to make provision for an aging population, whereas the other groups are characterized by a much younger age (Table 4-2).

Table 4-2. Percent of Population by Racial Group and Age

Age in Years	African	Asian	Colored	White
0-14	41	32	36	27
15-59	54	63	59	59
60-74	4	4	4	9
75+	1	1	1	5

Source: National Health and Population Development Epidemiological Comments, 1987

Life expectancy for women is 55 years and for men is 52 years (Table 4-3). The birth rate for 1990 was 3201/1000 and the death rate was 909/1000. Such demographic factors suggest a need for health programs aimed at interventions related to an expanding ill-educated younger population and a growing dependency in the aging groups.

Table 4-3. Life Expectancy at Birth by Population Group 1985

Population Group	Male (years)	Female (years)
African	55	61
White	68	76
Colored	58	66
Asian	64	71

Source: Center for Epidemiological Research, 1986.

THE HEALTH CARE SYSTEM, FINANCING AND UTILIZATION

The Health Care Delivery System

There are a total of 737 hospitals throughout South Africa. Each hospital is classified by ownership. Provincial hospitals are operated by one of the four authorities in the province ('non-home-land') area of South Africa; homeland hospitals are controlled by one of the authorities in the independent and self-governing home-lands; industrial hospitals owned and run by large industries; agricultural or mining corporations; province-aided private hospitals mainly in the Cape Province, provide care to non-private patients.

The current health care system in South Africa is maldistributed, poorly funded, uncoordinated, fragmented, duplicative, and discriminatory on a racial basis. The care is hospital based and supported by very poorly developed ancillary services. The present structure of the health service in South Africa dates back to the passing of the Public Health Act of 1919. The central government controls a minority of hospital services, including a number of tuberculosis institutions and mental hospitals. Most of the curative services, particularly the hospitals, fall under the control of the different provincial administrations. The central government is also responsible for the public health measures with the exception of the environmental controls, social health services, and control of communicable diseases. These are delegated to the local authorities in the provinces. Some private organizations, such as the Chamber of Mines, supplement the financial support for the hospitals that were owned by missions. When the mission hospitals were taken over by the central governments and the governments of black homeland in 1973, there were approximately 133 mission hospitals with a total of 34,000 beds. The hospitals had provided a valuable contribution through the century, had employed about 270 doctors and 1,880 registered nurses, and had provided training for 4,000 nurses.

South Africa currently spends approximately 5.9% of the GNP on health. The GNP per capita for the country is US $2,240. However, the GNP per capita conceals maldistribution of earnings. And these national figures conceal wide variations between geographical, social, economic, and racial sectors. Exact estimates are not available at national, regional and local levels for the percentage of national health expenditure devoted to preventive and promotive services. There is a need for a review of health expenditure accounting in order to obtain accurate data for future health-planning purposes. Some institutions provide private health insurance for their employees. South Africa does not have a national health insurance program although some recommendations for such have been submitted to the central government.

Of all the health care providers, nurses constitute the largest cadre (Table 4-4). Selected health indicators are presented in Table 4-5. The segregation of medical and social services according to population groups in South Africa is unique in the world. The incredible misuse of money and resources that result from the duplication of health services can only be explained by a system that perpetuates discrimination in both quantity and quality of health and welfare provided for Whites and for Africans. In 1987 there were 737 hospitals and 1,657 health centers and clinics in South Africa. The major hospitals are situated in the urban areas while the rural areas are deprived of readily available and adequate health facilities. The hospitals for Africans are overcrowded and understaffed.

Table 4-4. Health Personnel: 1986-1988

Health Personnel	1986	1987	1988
Medical practitioners {including specialists}	20,663	20,163	20,942
Dentists {including specialists}	3,486	3,408	3,581
Pharmacists	7,557	7,929	8,311
Nurses	87,235	134,552	140,718

Table 4-5. Health Indicators per 1000 People

Health Indicator	1986	1987	1988
Hospital beds	-	4.8	-
Medical practitioners	0.7	0.7	0.7
Nurses[a]	3.1	4.6	4.7

[a]1986 figures represent registered nurse, registered midwives/traditional birth attendants; 1987 and 1988 figures represent registered nurses, registered midwives/birth attendants, enrolled nurses, enrolled midwives and enrolled nursing assistants.

- **Physician Population Ratio by Race**

  1:333 for Whites
  1:730 for Asians
  1:12,000 for Coloreds
  1:91,000 for Africans
  1:1,540 for Overall Ratio
  Bantustans [Homelands]: Only 5% of doctors practice in the rural areas
  where 60% of the population lives.

- **Nurse Population Ratio**

  1:263 or 38 nurses to 10,000 people
  Total nurses: Whites 33.61%; Asians 2.04%; Coloreds 13.25%;
  Africans 51.09%

- **South African Nurses Council**

  1:416

- **World Health Organization recommendations for health indicators:**

  Nurse population ratio
  1:250 for First World Countries
  1:500 for Third World Countries

Health Service Utilization

The country's total fertility rate is 4.3 births per woman and the crude birth rate is 32.1/1000. The infant mortality rate (IMR) for the whole population was 64/1000 live births in 1985, which is high when compared with other countries. The IMR varies between population groups and is highest in Africans (males 73, females 68) and lowest in Whites (males 11, females 7). Adult mortality rates, as measured in terms of the chance of a 15-year-old dying before reaching the age of 60 ranges from 42.8% for African males and 29.4% for African females, to 21.8% and 11.5% for White males and females, respectively. The maternal mortality for the whole population is 5.5/1000 deliveries.

The maternal and neonatal services for the different population groups vary. Prenatal care for White women is provided by private medical practitioners for those women who are members of medical aid programs. Women who are not members of such programs generally attend the nearest hospital, where care is rendered by doctors and midwives employed by the provincial administration. Currently a very small percentage of all authorities offer antenatal and postnatal care for the White women. A limited number of White women utilize midwives in private practice. This approach to health care is new in South Africa. The service is compromised by these factors: a lack of support by medical personnel when complications arise; services rendered by midwives are not covered by medical aid programs; and most hospitals do not make beds available for births by midwives. Midwives are forced to offer their own homes or use the homes of their patients, which results in additional expenses.

The maternal and neonatal care services for the Africans are inadequate, inaccessible, and unacceptable. Owing to the inability of hospitals to meet the ever-increasing needs of the Black population in the Cape Peninsula and Soweto, obstetric midwife clinics have been established. At these clinics midwives offer antenatal, interpartum, and postnatal care, as well as postnatal follow-up services which constitute a major part of the midwife's task. In addition to keeping an eye on their patients' welfare, the midwives are on call for patients in large hospitals.

The clinics have a relatively easy access to medical care through the ambulance and flying squad services. Furthermore, they are organized so that a number of clinics are attached to a specific base-hospital to which all high-risk patients and patients with complications can be transferred while normal cases are handled by clinics. Although clinics are visited by doctors regularly, clinic-based midwives are given far greater responsibilities than those practicing in hospitals.

The primary advantage of the clinics is they bring obstetric services much closer to the patients while alleviating the pressure on hospitals. Referrals are followed at the clinics to ensure that patients with complications will be transferred to hospitals in good time in order to keep mortality figures as low as possible.

In the rural areas the satellite clinics are attached to the so-called "parent hospitals" and are responsible for obstetric services and extensive health services. Their functions are similar to urban-satellite clinics. Unfortunately, the communication system providing contact between the clinics and their base hospitals is not as effective as those used in urban areas. There is no telephone service; clinics cannot get in touch with their base hospital except by radio. Also, the lack of transport makes it difficult for the women who attended prenatal care to reach the clinic for delivery, especially at night. In order to overcome this problem, "waiting huts" have been erected on the clinic sites and women are encouraged to occupy these from their 28th week of pregnancy. Some of the women deliver at home with the assistance of a traditional birth attendant.

Between 1980 and 1982, many hospital studies ($N = 267$) were conducted throughout the country. Findings are presented in Tables 4-6 to 4-9. According to the researchers there was remarkable consistency in the major obstetric causes of death through a 25-year period (United Nations Population Studies, 1986). The most common cause of maternal death was hypertension, followed by hemorrhage, cardiac disease, sepsis, and pulmonary embolism. Avoidable factors involving medical attendants were present in 261 cases, whereas in 109 cases responsibility was ascribed to the patient (Table 4-8).

Table 4-6. Coverage of Maternity Care (%)

Area	Trained Attendant	Institutional Deliveries	Sample Size	Year
Cape Town	98	73	-	1981
Kwazulu (rural)	-	8	364	1983
Mosvold (rural)	-	54	212	1987

Table 4-7. Causes of Maternal Deaths

Causes	Number	%
Hypertensive disorders of pregnancy	224	30
Hemorrhage	125	18
Sepsis	106	14
Ruptured uterus	56	8
Embolism	48	7
Abortion	36	5
Complications of anesthesia	35	5
Ectopic pregnancy	5	1
Other direct obstetric causes	25	3
Direct causes (Total)	660	90
Indirect causes	61	8
Unrelated causes	13	2
Unknown	3	-
Total	737	100

Table 4-8. Classification of Factors

Factors	Number	%
Treatment given "too little too late"	87	11
Delay in consultation or transfer	25	3
Technical problems (surgical and anesthetic)		
Delay in diagnosis	24	3
Errors in diagnosis	11	1
Inadequate hospital facilities	11	1
Inadequate nursing care	5	0.5
Total	261	20

Table 4-9. Maternal Deliveries and Deaths by Race and Year

Year	Deliveries	Maternal Deaths	MMR (per 100,000 deliveries)
		Africans	
1975-77	11,554	8	69
1978-80	15,405	12	78
1981-83	21,159	11	52
		Coloreds	
1975-77	39,684	16	40
1978-80	42,291	14	33
1981-83	47,044	18	38
		Whites	
1975-77	3,708	1	27
1978-80	2,975	2	70
1981-83	2,514	0	-

Major Health Concerns of Women

Approximately 25% of women suffering from vesicovaginal fistulae (associated with obstructed and prolonged labor) experience amenorrhea after their pregnancies. Some women suffer from fistulae of the urinary tract. Women with this complication are unlikely to bear children unattended, they will find sexual intercourse impossible, and their social existence will be difficult because of the continuous urinary leak. Labor outcome of primiparae younger than 17 years is associated with assisted deliveries (vacuum extraction, forceps, cesarean section, and symphysiotomy). Adolescent pregnancy is on the increase in South Africa.

Perhaps the worst health problems for African women are gynecological. At worst, women find themselves unable to have children. An African woman is not accepted in the husband's family until she has a child. The reported cases of sterility are infection related. Infection can often be the result of venereal diseases, abortion, or infection from an intra-uterine device. The loop is a common contraceptive prescribed for Soweto women, including young girls.

Services for infertile women are few. The devastating experience of infertility is not a major concern for the health service planners. In fact, South Africa spends proportionately more on population control measures, than on any other health service. A 1983 report of the President's Council Science Committee on Demographic Trends suggested that population planning should be South Africa's highest national priority. The report said that South Africa will run out of water if the population continues to grow faster.

The incidence of syphilis in pregnancy is on the increase with an accompanying increase in perinatal morbidity and mortality. This increase is noted particularly in urban areas and developing communities and is probably related to socioeconomic factors. The failure to treat sexually transmitted diseases, such as syphilis and gonorrhea has been associated with higher rates of AIDS in Southern Africa (Table 4-10). Also, tuberculosis in any form is reported to be related to AIDS (Table 4-11).

Tuberculosis has been shown to decrease with a rising standard of living, better nutrition and improved housing, but in South Africa no attempt is made to tackle the problem from this angle. Instead, expensive measures are taken in the urban areas to treat the disease out of concern that whites might catch it through contact. Tuberculosis is increasing (Table 4-11). South Africa's overall immunization coverage (Table 4-12) is below average for developing countries where complete coverage increased from below 5% in 1974 to over 50% in 1986 (Global Status Report, 1987).

Table 4-10. Reported AIDS Cases as of January, 1991

Country	1986	1987	1988	1989	1990	Total
Botswana	11	25	22	29	0	87
Zimbabwe	0	119	202	1,311	3,617	5,249
Lesotho	1	1	3	6	0	11
Maputo	1	3	23	37	87	151
Namibia	4	15	43	127	122	311
South Africa	58	48	94	168	222	590
Swaziland	1	6	7	0	0	14
Tanzania	699	909	2,550	2,093	877	7,128

Source: WHO Vital Statistics: Southern Africa.

Table 4-11. Incidence of Notifiable Diseases, 1985 - 1988

Diseases	1985	1986	1987	1988
Typhoid fever	16.40	13.60	14.30	12.30
Meningococcal	1.90	1.80	2.30	3.10
Measles	55.40	43.90	72.30	46.40
Malaria	37.50	24.00	34.50	28.70
Tuberculosis	191.40	179.20	183.70	192.60
Viral hepatitis	5.50	4.90	5.20	6.20

Source: Statistical Abstracts, 1989.

Table 4-12. Immunization Coverage, 1984

Vaccine	% Fully Immunized	Notified Cases	Registered Deaths
Measles	39	14892	1095
Poliomyelitis	45	62	49
Diphtheria		43	9
Pertussis	44		18
Tetanus		260	53
BGG (TB)	63	54491	5773

EDUCATIONAL ACHIEVEMENT FOR WOMEN

The position of women in the ranks of professional workers reflects the status of women in South Africa, across the whole spectrum of color. The high proportion of women teachers is the result of a deliberate official policy: "in order to save money in teacher training and salaries, and also because women are generally better than men in handling small children." As in all areas, women are paid less than men. The available statistics shows some fluctuation in the ratio of female/male level of education (Table 4-13).

Table 4-13. Population by Age, Education, and Sex

Age	High School Male/Female	Junior Degree Male/Female	Senior Degree Male/Female
5+	3759/3776	2139/2212	175/95
15-19	774/785	339/377	124/147
20-24	565/589	433/446	139/162
25-34	969/929	571/557	59/37
35-54	1061/1007	578/567	729/296
55-64	223/242	129/141	172/6
65+	164/218	868/121	12/5

Source: Demographic Yearbook, 1990.

Women in general, both White and Black, are expected to operate in the home through parents' attitudes and expectations for their male and female children. In South Africa the lack of access to birth control and abortion leads to an extremely high rate of premarital pregnancy, resulting in a high school drop-out rate. The place assigned to the women in the social labor determines their access to education, and lack of access prevents them from obtaining any but the most rudimentary skills.

In the 1980s there were 97,300 African women and 79,880 African men classified as professionals. The overwhelming number of Black women in the professions are teachers or nurses. At the University level, only one-third of African students are women. In South Africa the lines of racialism and sexism converge. African people, both men and women, are educated within the "Bantu Education" based on the ideology of apartheid. The literacy rate (15 years and older) for the various groups has been estimated at: 98% for Whites; 50% for Africans; 75% for Colored; and 85% for Asians.

ECONOMICS

Official statistics recorded about a third of South African adult women as gainfully employed in 1988. Black women with no particular training, but in need of income, find jobs by visiting factories and reading the notices or just hanging around a factory until finding someone to ask. Very few women find employment through newspaper advertisements or the labor bureaus. Tables 4-14 through 4-18 address economic issues related to South African Women, including occupational status, percentage of economically active women, average wage by industry, and percentage of incomes below the subsistence level for a family of six.

Table 4-14. Occupational Status of Black Women (%)

Job status	Asian	African	Colored	All
Semi-professional	8.5	18.7	12.7	15.8
Sales and clerical	36.4	10.9	18.4	15.6
Skilled	1.5	1.8	4.2	2.5
Semi-skilled	42.6	23.7	39.3	30.5
Unskilled	10.7	44.7	25.2	35.3

Source: National Survey, N. 14, April, 1981.

Table 4-15. Occupation of Economically Active Women, 1921 and 1980 (%)

Occupation	Year	African	White	Colored	Asian
Agriculture	1921	88.4	4.8	5.5	40.9
	1980	15.8	0.6	8.6	0.6
Service	1921	10.2	18.3	84.9	27.0
	1980	42.4	5.6	32.1	7.2
Sales/clerical	1921	0.0	8.8	1.0	40.8
	1980	6.9	65.4	22.2	44.8
Professional	1921	0.1	20.8	1.3	0.1
	1980	5.5	21.9	21.9	5.5
Production	1921	0.0	9.6	1.8	3.2
	1980	10.7	2.8	26.6	39.7

Source: Figures for 1921 from South African Office of Census and Statistics; Figures for 1980 from the South African Statistics 1982.

Table 4-16. Economically Active Populations by Race and Sex, 1980

Race	African	White	Colored	Asian
Male	3,822,860	1,274,380	572,700	190,000
Female	1,754,480	630,680	355,080	65,820
Total	5,577,040	1,906,060	927,780	255,820

Source: Social Characteristics Report, Republic of South Africa, Central Statistics Service .

Table 4-17. Women's Average Monthly Income in Rand by Race and Industry

Industry	African	Asian	Colored	White
Food	196	385	290	993
Textile	209	362	263	1093
Clothing	120	210	197	935
Commerce/wholesale	245	564	338	1101
Commerce/retail	179	351	243	594

Source: Survey of Race Relations in South Africa—1982.
1 Rand = US $0.30.

Table 4-18. Percentages of Incomes and Earnings Below Minimum Subsistence Level for Family of Six, 1983

Race	Wives	Husbands	Family
African	94.5	87.6	80.3
Asian	86.7	75.6	66.5
Colored	42.7	38.3	42.3
Total	83.1	74.1	68.2

Source: National Manpower Surveys, 1983.

Women's entry into wage labor is restrained on the one hand by the reluctance of parents and husbands to release them from the home, and on the other, by the reluctance of the bosses to admit them onto the factory floor. The final "liberator" from these restrictions is economic pressure. Economic necessity compels the family to release the women from the home, and economic development forces bosses—who lose male labor to other, more lucrative sectors of industry and commerce—to employ them. The attitude of management to the employment of women is a crucial factor in determining their position in commerce and industry.

Women are most generally engaged in unskilled and semi-skilled jobs; Black women in a multi-racial system are most affected. This makes Black women more vulnerable to retrenchment due to mechanization and recession. The general thesis holds that they are the last to be hired—employed only when the men do not want the jobs—and the first to be fired when a scarcity of jobs develops due to fluctuations in the economy. Women are, in this context, a reserve army of laborers, finding employment during periods of economic expansion and being put out of work when the company sinks.

South African labor laws prohibit discrimination by sex in the employment sector; legislation "protecting" women from shift work was eliminated in 1983. Nonetheless, some factories still pay unequal wages to their male and female employees. It is noted that the Machinery and Occupational Safety Act and Mine's Works Act of 1983, and the Workmen's Compensation Act of 1941, regulate health hazards and accidents in the workplace. However, industries can be exempted from complying with the basic health and safety requirements. The women in the workplace have little consciousness of the health hazards they suffer or their rights to lay claim in the event of an accident.

With help from the trade unions, women are being considered for paid maternity leaves and job security. The Provident Fund of the Clothing Industry (Natal) offers pension benefits and the Industrial Council regulates holidays. Some workers are allowed sick leave up to 8 days a year. An appointed doctor and nurse are made available by the Sick Benefit Fund controlled by the

Industrial Council. The women are not actively involved in decision-making about retirement plans and they are not represented in the Wage Board.

Pension applications are processed in Pretoria and take between six months and a year to finalize. African widows do not qualify for maintenance grants in rural areas, although such grants are available to widows of other groups. Maximum monthly income for Africans in 1984 was R65 in comparison to R166 for Whites. Pensioners living in urban areas, outside of the bantustans, who wish to qualify must provide their living lawfully. They must produce documentary proof of age, which many old people are unable to do.

FAMILY STRUCTURE

Africans in both towns and country may choose to marry according to general South African law—common law—or according to traditional law—customary union. Marriage by common law is more usual in the towns; most Africans in the bantustans marry according to customary union. To enter into a customary union one must have parental consent and such marriages are validated by *lobolo* [dowry]. *Lobolo* was one of the means whereby women were under the dominion of men in traditional society. *Lobolo* is fading with the feminist movement in South Africa.

Under common law, married women's rights over children and property depend on the choice made by the marriage partners. The marriage can be legalized by what is called "community of property," or by the exclusion of community of property through legally drawn antenuptial contracts; or by marriage by common union. All of these ways incorporate disadvantages for women and involve their legal dependence. A new Matrimonial Property Act, which came into force in 1984, was lauded as a breakthrough for women. The new act abolishes marital power in marriages under common law. The power that made husbands the sole administrators of family property has been made to give joint administration to husband and wife. The mean age at first marriage is 22.8 years and the 1980 marital status of Africans and Whites is depicted in Table 4-19.

Table 4-19. Marital Status of Africans and Whites: 1980

Race	Total	Married	Unmarried
African	8,227,680 (100%)	1,917,280 (23%)	5,491,680 (76%)
White	2,262,700 (100%)	1,033,640 (46%)	954,420 (54%)

Source: Official 1980 Census Figures.

In town and country today, South Africa teaches potent lessons about the meaning of the family, patriarchy, and the exploitation of women. The illusion persists that the individual family is the basic economic unit of society. The conventional morality relating to the family, piously upheld by the state, by its propaganda, by its religious institutions, by its laws and its codes of ethics, is unrelated to reality. The establishment of bantustans, restrictions on women entering the towns, mass population removals, harsh laws relating to movement and work, and most of all, the spread of migrant labor, are all factors which have had a devastating effect upon human relationships as expressed in terms of marriage and the family.

Even with the legal rights to reside in towns, Black women live under the strains of great insecurity. Their legal status may be rescinded on a large variety of pretexts. A women must avoid the misfortune of being left without a husband whether through desertion, divorce, or death. She often loses her home as well as her husband. A divorced woman may be given permission to stay in her home only if she was not the guilty party in the divorce suit, and has been granted custody of the children; if she qualifies in her own right to remain in town; if she can pay the rent; and if her former husband has agreed to vacate the house. If he has remarried immediately, he may choose to remain in the house with his new wife. A woman who has no husband must avoid conduct which will lead an urban authority to hold her presence as "detrimental to the maintenance of peace and order" and therefore make her liable to removal.

SEXUALITY

Women need to be able to control their own fertility. But when birth control becomes population control, as it has in South Africa, it acquires a new significance. The White attitude to birth control is conditioned by racialist beliefs, and this found expression of the "haves" and "have-nots," the former group being intelligent, with a sense of responsibility and civilization; the latter lacking responsibility and "breeding recklessly."

In accordance with the Family Planning Association, contraception is theoretically free and available to all women (Table 4-20). But availability is dependent on access to clinics and despite the fact that there are 3,000 such clinics, women in remote rural areas are less likely to have either such access or the means to travel to the nearest clinic. Other factors associated with resistance to contraception were objections on religious, moral, and medical grounds for both White and Black people.

Table 4-20. Percentage of Contraceptives Used by Racial Groups, 1983

	Type of Contraceptive			
Race	Pill	Injectables	IUD	Total
African	38	59	3	100
Colored	45	54	1	100
Asian	80	17	3	100
White	77	19	4	100

Source: Family Planning Progress Report,1983.
Note: These figures exclude those women who get their contraceptives from private doctors.

The use of contraceptives amongst the Blacks is compounded by the fact that women fear anger from their men if their use of contraceptives is discovered, and many women are unable to obtain information about contraception because clinics would insist on the man's consent. South Africa was one of the testing grounds for injectable contraceptives. Experience both in South Africa and in other countries shows that women do want to know about conception control, and readily accept it when women's organizations or local midwives give the instructions. There is no simplistic answer to the problem of conception control; medical, religious, moral, and cultural factors, and standards of living play a part in forming attitudes. But the issues could only be resolved in a society that would give women status, education, and health facilities. According to a report from Health Statistics 1990, the coverage of usage for the Africans is 45% , Coloreds 60%, Asian 63% and Whites 66%. Abortion is virtually illegal in South Africa, although the Abortion and Sterilization Act of 1975 legalized abortion in certain closely controlled situations: if there is a threat to the permanent mental or physical health of the mother or child; if pregnancy is a result of rape or incest; or if the mother is an imbecile. The year after the introduction of the Act over 100,000 backyard abortions were still performed, while the majority of medical abortions were obtained by Whites (Abortion Reform Group, 1976).

Information about illegal abortions is difficult to obtain, but there are some indications. Approximately 25% of all bed space in gynecological wards in South Africa is occupied by women suffering from complications following back-street or self-induced abortions. Incomplete abortions are a leading cause of death in these units. The Center for Applied Social Sciences in Natal estimated that in 1970 alone, approximately 141,800 Black women and 17,800 White women resorted to abortion. Some women have traveled to Lesotho where a doctor from South Korea performed abortions. Baragwanath Hospital (Soweto, Johannesburg) runs two special wards on weekends to treat incomplete abortions. The Groote Schuur Hospital in the Cape was forced to support a special septic abortion unit which had the highest bed occupancy and highest patient turnover of any ward in the hospital. The King Edward VIII Hospital in Natal treated over 4,000 septic abortion cases in 1972.

VIOLENCE AGAINST WOMEN

Spouse abuse is associated with the men who work under conditions of exploitation which, because of their lack of political power and their exclusion from collective bargaining, are often beyond their control. It is the women who bear the brunt of the frustration and aggression that their husbands are powerless to express within the workplace. In South Africa, wife- and child-beating is as common as rape. Sexual aggression is, in a situation such as this, a more or less immutable fact of life.

Also, the overcrowding, crime, poverty, and increasing unemployment that are the features of township life impose massive strains on individuals. The family functions to absorb expressions of anger that are not allowed elsewhere. Often, men have had a hard day somewhere, get drunk, and take out their frustrations on wives and children. Battery and alcoholism are the most common results in this situation. In Soweto, 60% of children are born to unmarried women, and while parents may often marry after a child is born, more women are choosing not to marry.

It is extremely difficult to obtain accurate figures on the incidence of rape in South Africa. By far the largest number of rapes take place against Black women in the violent and degraded conditions in the urban townships where the police are more concerned with the suppression of resistance and the enforcement of apartheid than with crime prevention. Many cases go unreported and those cases reported may not be dealt with seriously by police.

According to reports, it is stated that in South Africa the estimate of reported cases is only one in twenty; and rape has the lowest conviction rate of any crime of violence in the country. A "Rape Crisis" report from Cape Town reported 41,341 men prosecuted for rape in a 4-year period. Of these, 22,408 were convicted and 19 were sentenced to death. The youngest rape victim was 3, the eldest 70. There were 41 cases of children under 17. The rape of a White woman is a serious crime that can result in a death sentence. In reported cases police themselves are frequently involved in the rape of a Black woman. As in other countries, humiliating police interrogation, unsympathetic medical examinations, and harassment by lawyers discourage women from proceeding with charges of rape. To this must be added the context of blatant racial prejudice, often expressed openly in obscene language by the police towards black women. Some women do not report rape because in some cases the rapist is known to the victim. Working women have reported sexual harassment and rape from management and male co-workers.

Harassment to women prisoners is compounded by separation from their children and uncertainty about their fate. Women have been prosecuted on a wide variety of political charges reflecting the range of their involvement in the struggle against apartheid, including treason, terrorism, sabotage, membership in or assistance to a banned organization, helping people to escape from the country, recruiting guerrillas, breaches of banning orders, and similar charges. Among those who are serving or have served jail sentences are women of all colors, ages, and religions. There are young girls, mothers, and grandmothers, some over 70 years of age.

Information on the conditions and treatment of women political prisoners is scarce, but the experiences of individual women prisoners indicate that their conditions may in some respects be even harsher than those endured by male political prisoners. Their isolation from the outside world is accentuated by the difficulties and obstruction which relatives face in locating and visiting them in prison. Women prisoners are not allowed to study throughout their sentence. Newspapers are denied to all women prisoners and letters do not reach them. The only reading material made available is the Bible.

WOMEN'S STRENGTHS AND POLITICAL PARTICIPATION

Women's political and social organizations cannot be addressed without discussing the problems and disabilities that apartheid inflicts on the whole black population. Also, it is not possible to assess the women's political activities and struggles without surveying the general struggle for liberation.

Women's organizations have always operated within the framework of the political resistance movements because women clearly understand that the reforms they need are dependent upon a restructuring of the state itself. Without the women's activities in the liberation struggle, the campaigns could not have taken place. In South Africa, women are not asking for women's rights but a combined fight against the system. Both white and black women are oppressed by leadership that is dominated by men. The most oppressed and deprived women are the 5 million now living in *bantustans*, trapped by the merciless apartheid system.

The trade union movement—the organizations through which workers state their demands, fight for basic rights, fight to improve wages and working conditions—does not fully appreciate the issues which affect women workers. The number of South African women who are members of organized trade unions is still small. Heightened political struggles in the community in the 1980s is reflected in the increased politicization of Black nurses. Apart from the equalization of pay, since 1991 wage bargaining machinery and compulsory arbitration were introduced for nurses and all references to racial discrimination being dropped from the South African Nurses' Association's constitution since 1991. Examples of other women's trade unions, political organizations, campaigns, and demonstrations include the following:

- **Trade Unions**

  The National Union of Textile Workers
  Federation of the South African Trade Unions
  The Food and Canning Worker Union
  Sweet Food and Allied Workers Union
  Transport and General Workers Union

- **Political Organizations**

  Federation of South African Women
  Natal Indian Women's Congress
  African National Congress Women's League
  Women for Peace
  United Democratic Front
  South African Domestic Workers Association
  United Women's Organization
  Black Sash
  Black Women's Federation

- **Campaigns in Which Black Women Have Participated**

  Orange Free State Women's Anti-Pass Campaign, 1913
  The Defiance of Unjust Laws Campaign, 1952
  Pretoria Anti-Pass Campaign, 1956-1957
  The Sharpeville Massacre, 1956
  The Riot Uprising, 1976

- **Other Demonstrations by Women**

  Demonstration in Support of Treason Trial, 1956
  Protest of Beerhalls at Cator Manor, 1959
  Demonstration at Mandela Trial, 1962
  Protest against Tricameral Parliament, 1983
  Rally of FSAW, 1984
  Rent Increase, 1985

South African women are not indifferent to the feminist movements of other countries, and the literature of feminism has given impetus to research into the history and activities of women, into the lives of women today, and into areas that have never been investigated before. The activities reveal circumstances, beliefs, and changing attitudes that make it possible to open the way for a greater participation of women in the struggle for freedom, as well as uncovering the past history of women's struggles.

CONCLUSION

Using surveys and indirect demographic research and underreporting health problems of Blacks in South Africa make the quality of vital and medical statistics unreliable. Promoting basic health and preventing diseasesshould replace hospital-based curative services. The challenge that health services currently face is to have to deal simultaneously with poverty-related diseases, chronic degenerative diseases, infections, trauma, and sexually-transmitted diseases. The challenge can be achieved through a comprehensive primary health care approach.

REFERENCES

AbouZahr, C., & Royston, E. (1991). *Maternal mortality: A global factbook.* Geneva: World Health Organization.

Bair, F. E. (Ed.). (1991). *Countries of the world and their leaders: Yearbook 1991.* Detroit: Gale Research Inc.

Benatar. R. (1990). A unitary health service for South Africa. *South African Journal of Medicine, 77,* 441-447.

Bernstein, H. (1985). *For their triumphs and for their tears: Women in apartheid South Africa.* London: International Defence and Aid Fund for Southern Africa.

Bradford, H. (1992). *Herbs, knives and plastic: 150 years of abortion in South Africa.* Paper presented at a women's symposium in London.

Cadler, P. W. (1971). *Modern health service in South Africa.* London: Struik (Pty) Ltd.

Catholic Institute for International Relations. (1985). *South African women on the move: Vukani makhosikazi.* London: Zed Books Ltd.

Cheater, A. (1974). A marginal elite? African registered nurse in Durban, South Africa. *African Studies, 33,* 3.

Flynn, D. K. (1992). *Building or burning bridges?* A report from the 1992 Women in Africa and African Diaspora Conference, Nigeria, Africa.

Friedland, I., et al., (1992). AIDS—The Baragwanath experience, Parts I, II, III, & IV. *South African Journal of Medicine. 88,* 86-102.

Hansen, T. K. (1984). Negotiating sex and gender in urban Zambia. *Journal of Southern African Studies, 10,* 219-238.

Jacobson, J. (1992). Improving women's reproductive health. *State of the World,* 1992, 83-99.

Klopper, M., et al., (1989). A methodology for resource allocation in health care for South Africa, Parts I, II, & III. *South African Journal of Medicine, 76,* 209-210; *77,* 453-458.

Kollstedt, E., & Bergstrom, S. (1991). Family planning and race in South Africa. *AIDS Watch.* (2nd Quarter) p 9.

Laidler, P. W., & Gelfand, M. (1971). South Africa: Its medical history. Cape Town: Gothic Printing Co., Ltd.

Lempert, L. (1986). Women's health from a women's point of view: A review of the literature. *Health Care for Women International, 8,* 255-275.

Mahler, H. (1981). Health 2000: The meaning of "Health for All by the Year 2000." *World Health Forum, 2,* 5-22.

Marks, S. (1987). Not either an experimental doll. *The separate worlds of three South African women.* London: The Women's Press, Ltd.

McAllister, P. A. (1980). Work, homestead and the shades: The ritual interpretation of labor migration among the Gcaleka. In P. Mayer (Ed.), *Black villagers in an industrial society.* New York: Oxford University Press.

Meer, F. (1990). *Black woman worker: A study in patriarchy and woman production in South Africa.* Natal: Madiba Publication.

Mella, P. (1986). Effects of educated professionals on the health and care of women in Tanzania. *Health Care for Women International, 8,* 239-248.

Morgan, R. (1984). South Africa (Republic of South Africa). In *Sisterhood is Global.* Garden City, NY: Anchor Books/Doubleday.

Population Crisis Committee. (1988). Country rankings of the status of women: Poor, powerless and pregnant. *Population, 20.*

Qunta, C. N. (1987). *Women in South Africa.* London: Allison & Busby Ltd.

Ramphele, M. (1989). The dynamics of gender politics in the hostels of Cape Town: Another legacy of the South African migrant labor system. *Journal of the Southern African Studies, 8,* 393-414.

Royston, E. (1991). *Maternal mortality: A global factbook.* South Africa. Geneva: World Health Organization.

Schuster, I. (1981). Perspectives in development: The problem of nurses and nursing in Zambia. *African Women in the Development Process.* London: Frank.

Seager, J., & Olson, A. (1986). *Women in the world: An international atlas.* New York: Simon & Schuster.

Statistical Abstract. (1989). *South Africa, Transkei, Ciskei, Bophutatswana and Venda population report.* Pretoria.

United Nations. (1991). *The world's women 1970-1990: Trends and statistics* (Social Statistics and indicators, Series K, No. 8). New York: United Nations Publications.

Uys, L., Uys, H., & Kotze, W. (1991). *State of the art of nursing: A centenary publication.* Pretoria: South African Nursing Association.

Walker, C. (1991). *Women and resistance in South Africa.* New York: Monthly Review Press.

Women 2000. (1992). Women in development. *United Nations Population Fund: Incorporating women into population and development, 1,* 1-20.

World Bank. (1992). *World development report 1992: Development and the environment.* Oxford: Oxford University Press.

Americas

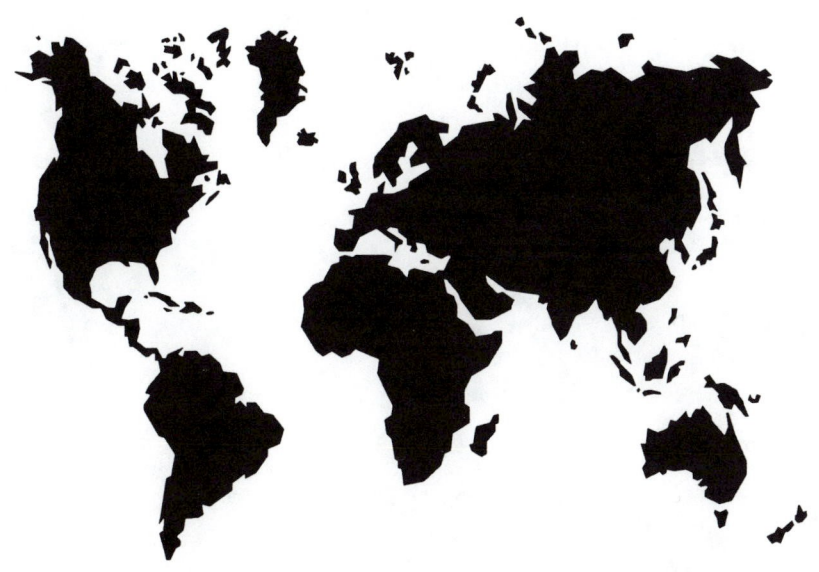

Brazil
Canada
United States

5

Women's Health Status in Brazil: The State of São Paulo and Ribeirão Preto Region

Collaborating Centre for Development of Nursing Research
Campus de Ribeirão Preto
University of São Paulo at Ribeirão Preto, College of Nursing

Maria Solange Guarino Tavares and Antonieta Keiko Kakuda Shimo

INTRODUCTION

The data for this chapter came from the 1987 Annual Statistical Report of the Brazilian Institute of Geography and Statistics (IBGA) and from other publications from the 1980s. The report does not include data from the 1991 Brazilian Population Census since the census was unpublished at the time this manuscript was written. Some population authorities have suggested that the rate of urbanization in Brazil will be higher in the recent data than the original projections based on 1980 census data.

POPULATION DISTRIBUTION

The geographical area of Brazil is 8,511,965 square kilometers with a population of 119,002,706 in 1980. A population census was not undertaken in 1990.

The results of the census taken in 1991 are expected to be published by June of 1992. Table 5-1 shows the population distribution by sex and color in 1980. The native Brazilian population is a mixture of black, white, and indigenous populations. Table 5-2 shows the female distribution of the population according to age groups in 1985. Women constitute roughly 50% of the population until age 65 when the percentage begins to exceed that of men. The female Brazilian population is almost evenly split between urban (51%) and rural (49%) areas.

Table 5-1. Population Distribution by Sex and Color

Color	Male (%)	Female (%)
White	56.0	56.9
Black	7.4	7.2
Brown	35.9	35.3
Total	100.0	100.0

Source: Brazilian Institute of Geography and Statistics (IBGE) National Household Sample Poll (PNAD), 1982.

Table 5-2. Female Distribution of Brazilian Population by Age Groups

Age (Years)	Female Population		Total Population	
	Number	(%)	Number	(%)
0-14	23,481	(35)	47,879	(37)
15-49	33,634	(51)	66,953	(50)
50+	9,155	(14)	17,488	(13)
Total	66,270	(100)	132,320	(100)

DEMOGRAPHIC PROFILE

Brazil's government is a presidential democracy. The country's social and economic system is based on the capitalistic economic model. Portuguese is the language spoken throughout Brazil. Table 5-3 shows the literacy rates for the population, by age and sex. Prior to age 30, women are slightly more literate than men, then the trend reverses with men slightly more literate than women. Table 5-4 reports female literacy rates by place of residence (urban and rural), and age group.

Table 5-3. Female Literacy Rates in Brazil, by Age, 1985

Age Group	Female (%)
5-6	7
7-9	57
10-14	85
15-19	91
20-24	90
25-29	88
30-39	82
40-49	72
50-59	63
60+	47

Source: PNAD, 1985.

Table 5-4. Female Literacy Rates by Age and Area, 1985

Age Groups	Urban	Rural
7-29	89.8	68.0
30+	76.0	45.4

The 1987 projected infant mortality rate for 1990 (Brazilian Annual Statistical Review) is 63.32 per 1,000 live births. In the decade of 1970-1980, the death rate in the Brazilian population was 87.88 per 1000, with a death rate of 85.19 per 1000 in the urban population and 92.90 per 1000 in the rural population. In 1986, the death rate in the state of São Paulo was 74.65 per 1000. The principal causes of death in the Brazilian state capitals in 1984 is presented in Table 5-5.

In 1980, the projected life expectancy for the Brazilian population was 65.5 years for women and 61.3 years for men. Table 5-6 reports the infant, neonatal, and postneonatal mortality rates, and the crude death and birth rates in Brazil for the years 1989 and 1990.

The Brazilian Health Care System

The health sector includes both private and governmental services. Government resources are centralized at the federal, state, and municipal levels, but health care administration has recently been delegated to the municipal level. The government is the major health care employer and consumer. In addition to

Table 5-5. Principal Causes of Female Death in Brazilian State Capitals, 1984 (Rate x 100,000)

Cause	Death Rate	Proportionate Mortality (%)
Malignant neoplasms	73	14
Cerebrovascular disease	70	13
Ischemic heart disease	55	10
Diseases of the pulmonary circulation and other heart disease	43	8
Perinatal causes	36	
Acute respiratory infections	35	6
Intestinal infections	28	5
Diabetes Mellitus	19	3
Hypertensive disease	16	3
Vascular disease	13	2
Nutritional deficiencies	12	2
Automobile traffic accidents	10	2
Chronic obstructive pulmonary disease	10	2
Accidents (other than traffic)	10	2
Diseases of the urinary system	8	2
Congenital malformation	8	1
Nonspecific acute edema and other pulmonary diseases	8	1
Septicemia	7	1
Appendicitis, abdominal hernia and peritoneal and abdominal complications	6	1
Chronic liver disease	5	1

Table 5-6. Mortality and Birth Rates in Brazil, 1989-1990

Year	IMR[a]	NMR[b]	PNM[c]	CDR[d]	CBR[e]
1989	21.87	13.96	7.91	5.06	18.49
1990	21.94	16.39	5.55	6.35	17.92

[a]IMR = Infant Mortality Rate (CIS-SEADE) and SMS-RP.
[b]NMR = Neonatal Mortality Rate (CIS-SEADE) and SMS-RP.
[c]PNM = Postneonatal Mortality Rate (CIS-SEADE) and SMS-RP.
[d]CDR = Crude Death Rate (CIS-SEADE) and SMS-RP.
[e]CBR = Crude Birth Rate SMS-RP.

providing services, the government purchases health care services from the private sector for care of individual consumers. Thus, the Brazilian health care system is a mixed private and public system. The government public health system has traditionally offered basic health care services through a network of basic health care units (health posts) and health centers. These primary level services are integrated into a regionalized hierarchical network, which is known as the Unified Health System (SUS) and has been implanted in the majority of Brazilian municipalities in recent years. Health care services are also offered by private enterprise; however, government financing for health care services is accomplished through the following mechanisms:

- The federal budget for health prioritized funding of public health measures and epidemiological surveillance.
- The National Social Security and Social System (INSS)
- State and Municipal Health Department

In practice, there is little if any evidence that Primary Health Care has been integrated into the national health care system, in either the more developed or lesser developed areas of Brazil. What is most evident at all levels of health care services is the provision of health care based on emergency needs. In some parts of rural north and northeastern Brazil, lay midwives continue to provide health care to women and assist during labor and delivery and with the care of newborns. The percentage of women in various categories of health care workers is presented in Table 5-7.

Table 5-7. Percentage of Brazilian Health Care Workers Who Are Female, 1980

Professions	%
Physicians	21
Dentists	28
Pharmacists	38
Nurses	94
Nursing personnel	84
Non-nursing personnel	31

zilian Health Care Service

For each of the 5,000 Brazilian municipalities there are an average of 13 ·hospital health care establishments. Of these health care establishments, 16% Iealth Centers (CS), 47.6% are Health Posts (Psa), 4.5% are Medical Care (PAM), 24.1% are Polyclinics (POL) and 7.8% are Combination Units (both out-patient and in-patient) or Emergency Rooms (UM/PS). Overall, the public sector dominates the para-hospital sector of health care services.

Utilization of Health Care Services

In 1985 there were a total of 28,972 health care establishments in Brazil, of which 58.9% (17,076) were public institutions and 41.1% (11,896) were private services. The public health care services included 4,245 health posts (24.9%), 9,670 health centers (56.7%), 150 medical assistance posts (1.04%), 467 Emergency Room Services (2.7%), 1,002 Combination Units (5.8%) and hospitals. In the same year, the number of hospital beds was 532,283, of which 137,543 (25.8%) were in public institutions. A total of 13,138 of the public hospital beds were earmarked for obstetrics and gynecology. There are 394,740 (74.2%) hospital beds in private institutions, of which 44,002 (11.2%) were earmarked for obstetrics and gynecology.

The State of São Paulo had 16.6% of all the health care institutions in Brazil and 24.4% of all hospital beds. In 1985 The State of São Paulo had 4,808 health care establishments, of which 41.6% were public and 54.8% were private. There were 129,838 beds in the state, of which 15.5% were in public hospitals and 84.5% were in private institutions. In São Paulo, 1.143 (5.4%) of the public hospital beds were occupied by obstetrical and gynecological patients, whereas 10.7% (11,771) of the private hospital beds were occupied by the same specialties.

At the Municipal Health Department health posts in Ribeirão Preto in 1991 there were a total of 56,250 gynecological physicians visits and 26,808 obstetrical physicians visits, making a total of 83,058 visits in the area of women's health. The Municipal Health Department health post activities also include Child Health, Geriatric health, and Oral health. Roughly two-thirds of the population are covered for Polio, DPT, Measles, and BCG.

At the local level, 1991 data from Ribeirão Preto and the surrounding region show that the vast majority of births occur in hospitals, as well as a very high cesarean-section rate.

Education

According to the 1980 census data, the Brazilian population over age 5 was 102,579,006 persons, of which 68% (69,703,993) were considered literate, 31.9% (32,731,347) did not know how to read and write, and 0.1% (43,666) were undeclared as to literacy status. According to the IBGE 1987 Annual Statistical Report, the illiteracy rate of adults over 15 years of age in urban areas was 13.89% compared to the illiteracy rate of 38.9% in rural areas.

Economic Considerations

The Brazilian Constitution of 1988 guarantees equal rights to males and females concerning legal rights, inheritance rights, and access to employment, trade, or profession. Fifty-six percent of the population age 10 and over is considered economically active. Within this group, 66.5% are male and 33.5% female. Of the population considered not to be economically active, 26.7% are male and 73.3% are female. Employment rates by sex and age group in 1985 are shown in Table 5-8. Table 5-9 shows the distribution of employed people by sex and type of employment in 1985.

Table 5-8. Employment Rates by Sex and Age Group, 1985

Age Group	Female	Male
10-14	12.24	26.52
15-19	41.74	73.33
20-24	50.13	92.50
25-29	48.46	97.16
30-39	49.71	97.44
40-49	43.53	93.95
50-59	30.30	80.79
60+	10.42	45.24

Source: IBGE; PNAD 1985.

Table 5-9. Percentage Distribution of Employed Persons by Sex, According to Branch of Employment, 1985

Branch of Employment	Female	Male
Agriculture	21.6	78.4
Basic industry	26.3	73.7
Civil construction	1.8	98.2
Other industry	10.2	89.8
Commerce	31.8	68.1
Service	64.5	35.5
Auxiliary service	28.2	71.8
Transportation and communication	7.8	92.2
Social	73.1	26.9
Public administration	25.5	74.5
Other activities	31.2	68.8
Total	33.3	66.7

Source: IGBE, PNAD 1985

Marriage and Family Structure

In Brazil, marriage is a civil institution, but the religious wedding ceremony may be recognized legally. The stable union between an unmarried couple may also be recognized by law. Equal legal rights are guaranteed to both husband and wife in the marriage contract. Divorce is legal in Brazil. Divorce can be granted after a legal separation of one year or more, or evidence of actual separation for two or more years. In 1980 the Brazilian census reported the following marital status for the population: single persons (21.0%), married persons (35.3%), separated (1.2%), legally separated or divorced (0.3%), widowed (3.0%), and undeclared (0.9%).

Breastfeeding Trends

The National Household Sample Poll (PNAD) of 1981 estimated that 88.4% of rural women and 85.4% of urban women initiate breastfeeding of their infants, and continue breastfeeding for an average of 12.3 weeks.

Sexuality

The Brazilian Constitution of 1988 allows for the utilization of family planning activities and choice of method by both men and women. According to the Constitution, it is the government's responsibility to provide educational and technical resources for the implementation of family planning, but any form of coercion on the part of private or governmental institutions is expressly prohibited. Although there are no legal restrictions concerning the women's liberation movement, there have been accusations of personal discrimination at the workplace or at home.

Abortion is illegal in Brazil but clandestine abortions are performed frequently throughout the country. Data concerning the occurrence of illegal abortions are not considered reliable since many abortions are reported as first trimester bleeding and diagnosed as spontaneous abortions. Although both abortion and permanent sterilization are prohibited by law, surgical sterilization of both females and males is openly practiced throughout the country. Female circumcision is not customarily practiced in Brazilian society.

The fertility rate in Brazil has shown a downward trend since 1970, as reflected by a rate of 5.7 (Brass method) in 1970 and a lower rate of 4.35 in 1980. The total fertility rate in 1984 was 3.53 with an urban rate of 3.03 and a rural rate of 5.32 (IBGE, Population Census and PNAD, 1984, Special Supplement on Fertility).

Women as Victims of Violence and Sexual Abuse

According to CHAUI, violence is considered an expression of force, domination, exploitation, and oppression manifest in asymmetrical social relationships, either in the area of social class or interpersonal relationship. The Police Department reported that violence against women and children in the Municipality of São Paulo from August to December of 1985 included 95.9% of the reported cased as violence against women and 4.5% against children and adolescents. In 85.5% of the cases the violence occurred between couples living together and in 10% of the cases violence occurred between people in other types of relationships (Table 5-10). Table 5-11 presents the incidents of violence according to type of abuse. As seen in the reports, 35% of the reported cases of violence were intentional bodily injury, 26.3% verbal abuse, and 25.9% threats. In 52.9% of the cases the assailant was identified as the victim's husband, 18.4% as her companion, 6.4% as her ex-husband, and 3.2% as her boyfriend (Table 5-12). Data for Tables 5-10 through 5-12 were registered at the Police Department for the Protection of Women in the Municipality of Sao Paulo in 1985.

Goldenberg et al. (1987) found that in 49% of the acts of violence between couples not living together, the woman was pregnant. Differing from cases of family conflict when the employed husband attacks his wife or companion, in these cases the abuse appears to be associated with poverty, unemployment, and delinquency.

Table 5-10. Incidents of Violence against Women, Children and Adolescents according to Type of Relationship

Types of Relationship	Percent
Incidents with women as victims	95.5
Between couples	85.5
At home	71.9
Outside the home	14.2
In other relationship	10.0
Family relations	3.2
Not family relations	6.8
Incidents with children and adolescents as victims	4.5
Family relations	2.0
Not family relations	2.5
Total	100.0

Source: CECF-SP/SEADE; Total number of cases: 2,037.

Table 5-11. Incidents of Violence against Women, Children and Adolescents according to Type of Assault

Type of Assault	Percent
Intentional bodily injury	35.1
Verbal abuse	26.4
Threat	26.0
Rape	3.9
Seduction	3.0
Slander	1.4
Assault on decency	1.0
All others	3.2
Total	100.0

Source: CECF-SP/SEADE; Total number of cases: 2,037.

Table 5-12. Incidents of Violence against Women, Children and Adolescents according to Type of Assailant

Type of Assailant	Percent
Husband	52.9
Companion	18.4
Ex-husband	6.4
Ex-companion	3.7
Boyfriend	3.2
Unknown person	2.1
Other male relative	1.8
Father	1.5
Acquaintance	1.3
Neighbor	1.1
All other	7.6
Total	100.0

Source: CECF-SP/SEADE;Total number of cases: 2,037.

Women's Movement

In São Paulo, the women's movements began in the 1970s. Initially these movements involved primarily professional and middle-class women. Eventually, mother's clubs and women's groups were formed in lower class neighborhoods, involving women in various social causes and issues.

The feminist groups became somewhat dispersed in the 1980s, and many feminists joined the Brazilian Democratic Movement (MDB), becoming involved in government party politics. A significant number of women participated in the Constitutional Assembly and presented proposals related to women's rights and women's health.

Women and Politics

The participation of women in political parties and campaigns has resulted in certain initiatives and proposals which have been incorporated by both state and federal governments. Examples of such initiatives are municipal and state commissions to deal with the feminine condition, the National Board of Womens' Rights, and the creation of police departments to deal with women's issues. In the health sector, the Program for Integrated Women's Health Care (PAISM) has been implemented in the public health service.

National women's organizations promote meetings, conferences and congresses for feminists, promoting the political and social involvement of women. Brazilian women have been encouraged to become more involved in their particular sphere of activity, and have done so in universities, neighborhood associations, and women's support groups. These women have had an important role as advocates for women's rights in general. They have also advocated for the creation of homes for abused women and for more dignity and respect in the provision of health care for all Brazilian women.

Other Aspects of Interest to Women's Health

There is a growing awareness of the need for obstetric nurses and midwives in Brazil. The following strategies are recommended for the implementation of change:

1. Deliveries are generally performed in hospitals by doctors in Brazil, ranging between 80 to 100% depending on the region of the country.

2. In some regions the incidence of cesarean delivery ranges between 70 to 90%.

3. Various factors influence this situation: specialized education of the doctor; technological advances in the area of obstetrics; larger fees for a cesarean delivery diminishing the value of a normal delivery; low salaries which oblige the doctor to have various places of employment.

4. Due to this situation, there is a national tendency to use the obstetric nurse or the midwife for deliveries as a strategy to decrease the frequency of cesarean deliveries.

5.　At the same time, discussions are occurring in Brazil about the necessity of the formation of the general nurse, abolishing the formation of a professional specifically trained in this area with the removal of training in obstetrics and the closing of schools of obstetrics, despite the fact that these schools are registered with MEC (Ministry of Education and Culture) as schools of nursing and obstetrics. With this, is the reality that few schools of nursing offer training in obstetrics, leading to a scarcity in the formation of the professional specialized in this area. (Approximately 1% are midwives according to the Federal Council of Nursing Census in 1988).

6.　There is a necessity to maintain trained personnel (24 hours a day) for the performance of normal deliveries in the hospital.

7.　Due to this, it is recommended that the nurse assists the mother during this period. Thus, there is a necessity of training nurses in obstetrics.

In the short term there should be recycling of practicing nurses, specialized courses in obstetrics, and greater emphasis on undergraduate education in obstetrical nursing. In the long term the National Health Program should stimulate the return of the professional midwives or obstetric nurses into women's health (PAISM), and train nurses at the graduate degree level who will be a multiplying agent.

6

Women's Health Status in Canada

Collaborating Centre for Nursing Development
McMaster University
School of Nursing

Andrea Baumann and Halina Connor

SYNOPSIS OF COUNTRY

(a) Area: Canada.
(b) Population: Total population: 26,832,700 (as of January 1, 1991); (102 females to every 100 males).
(c) Form of government: Parliamentary Democracy.
(d) Major health concerns: AIDS/maternal-infant mortality/chronic illness.

Demographics

(a) Language: French/English.
(b) Races: Multiethnic community.
(c) Other ethnic divisions; N/A.
(d) Data for literacy rates by gender and age is unavailable.
(e) Birth rates: 399,300 births in 1990, although the figure for births is expected to reach 404,000, an increase of approximately 3%.
(f) Death rates: 193,500 deaths in 1990.

(g) Infant mortality rates: 7 per 1,000 age 1-4 (0.4 per 100,000). Percentage of low income in neighborhood of residence is strongly and consistently related to measures of unfavorable birth outcomes. Based on data currently available for Canada, health problems of poor children begin before birth and place these children at greater risk for death, disability and other health problems throughout infancy, childhood and adolescence. Canada ranks seventh in the world for the lowest infant mortality.

(h) Life expectancy overall for men and women: women's life is 6.5 years longer than men's. On average, males live to age 72 and women live to age 78. Life expectancy at birth (in years): Males—73.6 versus females—80.4.

(i) Sex ratio at birth and at later ages: 102 females to every 100 males.

HEALTH CARE SYSTEM/FINANCING

Type of System

"Universal Health Care System"—Health Insurance Coverage for most medical expenses. There is universal unlimited access to health care. Health care is approximately 9% of the Gross National Product (GNP), with hospital care accounting for 40% of cost. Health care costs increased by 83.4% in constant dollars from 1975 to 1987 and increasing hospital costs accounted for the largest share of this increase.

Health Human Resources

There was one registered nurse for every 119 residents in 1990. The total number of registered nurses in the country was 256,145. Nearly 40% work part-time. Hospitals employ 73% of nurses, community health, 9%, and the remainder were employed in doctor's offices, educational institutions, and other employers. Fifteen percent of all nurses have a university degree. There are presently 55,000 physicians in Canada (GP & Specialists) and approximately 2,000 medical residents.

Health Services Utilization

Teenagers account for 5% of births overall. Of the 5%, 9% were from poor economic backgrounds. Among teenage women, the percentage of Small for Gestational Age, (SGA) births was 13%, compared to older women. Mothers from the poorest areas of Canada tend to be younger, of lower parity, frequently unmarried and are more apt to be born outside of Canada (Health Report, 1991a, 1991b). Teenage mothers are likely more than other mothers to live in poor areas, to be having a first child, to be unmarried and to have been born in Canada (p. 21). This is specifically related to urban versus rural areas. Poor children are less healthy than children of other Canadians. The differences in terms of excess mortality related to low income have narrowed some (1971).

Caesarean section rates have more than quadrupled in the last two decades in Canada. It has the second highest rate after the U.S.

EDUCATIONAL ACHIEVEMENT FOR WOMEN

In higher education, more women are enrolled than men in Canada at a ratio of 113 females to 100 men. At first level education (ages 5-12) the ratio is 93 females per 100 males. At second level education (ages 13-15) the ratio is 95 females per 100 males. At third level education (ages 17-23) the ratio is 113 females per 100 males.

ECONOMICS

(a) Percentage of women-headed households: 25%.
(b) Ages 15 and over: women economically active in 1990: 5,313,000.
(c) Economic activity rate in 1990: females (49%) and males (78%).
(d) Occupational groups (females/100 males):
Administrators, managerial workers: 54 females versus 100 males.
Clerical, sales, service workers: 178 females versus 100 males.
Production, transport workers laborers: 17 females versus 100 males.

FAMILY STRUCTURE

(a) Average household size: 2.8.
(b) Percent of women with children and no spouse: 25%.
(c) Percent of women living alone: 12%.
(d) Average age at first marriage: 23.1 (female) versus 25.2 (male).
(e) Total births per women in 1990: 1.7.
(f) Women currently married: 4.6%—age 15-19.
(g) Women currently married: 62%—age 25+.
(h) Percent of women 60 and not currently married: 51%.
(i) Percent of women ages 25-44 currently divorced: 5.4%.
(j) Women typically have their first child at 23 and their last at 30, for a span of seven years.
(k) Number of divorces in 1989: 80,736.

(l) Divorce rate per 100,000 population in 1989: 307.8.

(m) Divorce rate per 100,000 married women in 1989: 1,258.5.

Under the Divorce Act, a divorce could be obtained if either spouse had committed a 'matrimonial offense' such as adultery, physical or mental cruelty, or if the marriage had broken down permanently (1968). Under the 1985 Divorce Act, marriage breakdown is the sole ground for divorce. Four reasons for marriage breakdown are recognized, including separations for not less than one year, adultery, physical cruelty, and mental cruelty.

Custody of children: In 1989, there were 27,867 divorces involving custody orders granted under the 1985 Act. Of the 48,456 children affected, 74.2% were awarded to wives, 12.6% to husbands, 12.9% to joint custody, and fewer than 1% to a person other than the husband or wife.

SEXUALITY

There are no legalized practices of female circumcision nor restriction of movement within or across provinces. There are no contraception laws although there are some religions that do not encourage contraception (e.g., Catholicism). In 1989, there were 70,779 therapeutic abortions performed in Canadian hospitals which is an increase of 68% from the 66,251 performed in 1988. Of the 70,779 therapeutic abortions in 1989, 70,705 related to Canadian women and the remaining 74 were foreign women. For Canadian residents, the 1989 ratio for abortions performed in hospitals was 1.2 per 1,000 women ages 15-44, compared to a rate of 12.6 in 1988. Of the 70,705 women who obtained therapeutic abortions in hospitals, approximately 22% were below age 20, 54% between 20-29 years, another 22% between 30-39 years, and the remaining 2%, forty years and over. Over 53% had no delivery prior to the abortion, 19% had one previous delivery and 22% two or more deliveries. For the remaining 6%, the number of previous deliveries was not specified. About 8% of the women had at least one previous spontaneous abortion and 23% at least one previous induced abortion.

VIOLENCE AGAINST WOMEN

Sexual assault and rape: In Canada, women are about seven times more likely to be assaulted than men. The types of violence reported against women were homicide in the family, sexual assault and rape, and sexual harassment. Accurate indicators on domestic violence are often obtained from small studies and cannot be used to provide precise figures on the extent of violence against women, although they show that violence in the home is common and that women are most frequently the victims. There are protective measures used to assist abused women, including the police, shelters, non-governmental organizations, legal aid, financial assistance, and housing assistance.

WOMEN'S STRENGTHS

There are a variety of political and social organizations. There is a Status of Women division at the Federal and Provincial levels and a variety of municipal women's organizations, i.e., non-governmental and governmental.

POLITICAL PARTICIPATION OF WOMEN

Thirteen per cent of the population of women hold parliamentary positions in Canada. Women were granted the right to vote in Quebec in 1949, but in the rest of Canada it was in 1921. Years ago, women who were serving in the military or who had a close male relative serving in the military (father, husband, or son) were granted the right to vote at the federal level. Women were given the right to stand for election at the federal level 3 years later. Most women in government leadership are in such ministries as education, culture, social welfare and woman's affairs.

REFERENCES

1. Health Reports. (1992). Vol. 3, No. 1, Statistics Canada.
2. Health Reports. (1992). Vol. 3, No. 2, Statistics Canada.
3. 1991 Census of Canada, 1991.
4. The World's Women 1970-1990: Trends and Statistics, United Nations, New York, 1991.

7

Women's Health Status in the United States

Associated with The University of Illinois at Chicago
WHO Collaborating Centre

INTRODUCTION

The average woman in the United States is 34 years old. Around the middle of the next century, the average age of women will be 45 as the baby boomers (born 1946-1964) settle into later years. Of 100 women, 84 are white, 13 are black, 8 are Hispanic, and 3 are of other races. If the rates of birth, mortality, and net migration continue through the middle of the next century, 75 women would be white, 16 black, 17 Hispanic, and 9 of other ethnic backgrounds (Taeuber, 1991). Full-time, year-round female workers in the U.S. earn about 70% of the earnings of comparable male workers (Sidel, 1992).

The United States is an affluent industrialized nation, with the highest per capita health care expenditures in the world. However, women continue to lack essential preventive health care and suffer disproportionately from specific health problems. Three key factors shape women's health in the United States. First, as in many other countries throughout the world, generations of gender discrimination have meant that research and treatment have neglected women's unique health concerns. Second, women of color suffer double discrimination, as women and as members of minority ethnic groups. And finally, the lack of a national health program or universal health insurance has resulted in substantial inequality of health care by gender, race, and socioeconomic status. To understand the health care needs of women in the United States, this paper first describes the features of the U.S. health care system that affect women. Then the most important health needs of women are discussed, with the exception of maternal-child health needs discussed in Chapter 9.

THE UNITED STATES HEALTH CARE SYSTEM

The U.S. health care system is a combination of public and private efforts. It is pluralistic and complex and features large fiscal expenditures for health care delivery, which in 1991 were 14% of the Gross National Product (GNP). The health care system is governed in a highly decentralized manner through numerous state, county, and community entities, giving the system fairly permissive laissez-faire concepts throughout its health system (Roemer, 1991). Four major types of health programs operate to some degree in the United States: the private health care market, government health agencies, voluntary health agencies, and enterprises with health functions.

Currently, the U.S. health system is dominated by a private market. Ambulatory medical care (both general and specialist), dental care, medical and surgical services, pharmacy services, optical services, and fitting of prosthetic devices are services provided primarily by private practitioners. Personal preventive services are often financed by government or other organized entities, but a large share of its services are provided by private providers. Even when the financial support for health services is collectivized as in public or voluntary or in the tax-supported Medicaid program for the poor, the services are provided mainly through the private market. In essence, the responsible third party pays a private fee (Roemer, 1991).

The Department of Health and Human Services (DHHS) is responsible for most aspects of the nation's health and the administration of Social Security and public assistance programs. Other federal government departments that serve health functions include the Departments of Labor (Occupational Safety and Health Administration), Interior, Agriculture, Treasury (narcotic drug controls), Veterans Affairs, Defense, and Justice (Roemer, 1991).

Additional government agencies are involved with health at the state and local levels. Work-area inspections, worker compensation and vocational rehabilitation programs, public water supply, sewage disposal, and air pollution fall under the auspices of state control. In addition, special state authorities are generally concerned with the licensure and surveillance of nurses, physicians, pharmacists, and other health personnel. At the local level, boards and agencies monitor public schools, garbage disposal, mental health, and parks and recreation (Roemer, 1991).

Voluntary agencies raise funds to carry out programs for fighting certain diseases; focus on the health of certain population groups of concern, or certain types of health services such as visiting nursing care or blood donations. The disease-specific voluntary agencies that mobilize the interest and financial contributions of citizens are the most numerous (Roemer, 1991). Interestingly, the number of U.S. households that reported making charitable contributions to a health care organization increased from 28.2% in 1989 to 32.4% in 1990 (Data Watch, 1991).

Enterprises with health functions include large companies or mines with occupational health nurses and physicians and schools. Enterprises in isolated sites such as mines, railroad junctions, or lumber mills, occasionally operate comprehensive medical care programs for employees. Large industrial firms are required by law to protect employees from accidents and occupational diseases. Unfortunately, enforcement of the regulations may be weak (Roemer, 1991).

The U.S. health system has extensive buy poorly coordinated regulations and legislation. In 1952, the nongovernmental Joint Commission on Accreditation of Hospitals was organized; it is now the Joint Commission on Healthcare Organizations (JCAHO). The JCAHO accredits hospitals on a voluntary basis with 79% of U.S. hospitals currently accredited. JCAHO is recognized as the foremost evaluator of hospitals and home health care organizations in the U.S. (Pink, 1991). In addition, codes of ethics are established by professional organizations. Also, U.S. health insurance organizations set their own rules and regulations. Moreover, the judicial system provides regulation in the U.S. health care system. A patient who believes that a physician has caused undue harm may bring suit in a court of law. Most cases are settled out-of-court by the physician's insurance company. Lawsuits are costly. Therefore almost all physicians carry malpractice insurance (Roemer, 1991). In 1990, physicians reportedly paid 3.7% (about twice that in high-risk specialties of obstetrics, surgery, and anesthesiology) of their practice receipts in malpractice insurance (Special Report, 1992).

HEALTH PROFESSIONS

In 1990, there were 2,000,000 registered nurses (RNs), the largest group of health care providers in the U.S. About 94% of RNs are female. There are three levels of preparation for entry-level registered nursing practice: two years of community college preparation (Associate Degree—ADN); three years through a hospital-based program (Diploma); four years of university preparation (Bachelor of Science—BSN). Forty percent of all American RNs have ADN preparation, 25% have Diplomas, and 25% have BSN preparation (National League for Nursing, 1992).

In October 1990, the total number of nursing schools was 1470, essentially unchanged since 1983. There were 829 ADN programs, 489 BSN programs and

152 Diploma programs. From 1985 - 1990, there was an increase of 24% in enrollment of ADN programs, while Diploma and BSN programs decreased by 27% and 10%, respectively. The probable reasons for the increased number of ADN graduates is related to fewer educational requirements and relatively inexpensive tuition (National League for Nursing, 1992). The number of nursing schools exceeds the number of schools of medicine, osteopathy, podiatry, optometry, and dentistry combined (Bureau of Health Professions, 1990).

FUNDING OF THE U.S. HEALTH SYSTEM

The U.S. health care system funding sources are numerous and include the following:

1. Out-of-Pocket Expenditure is direct spending for health care which includes direct spending by consumers for all health care goods and services. This includes the amount not covered by insurance; the amount of coinsurance and deductibles required by private insurance companies and public programs, including Medicare and Medicaid; the payment to providers for services and goods that exceed the usual, customary, or reasonable charges paid by third parties.

2. Private Health Insurance includes traditional insurers such as commercial carriers Blue Cross and Blue Shield, and health maintenance organizations (HMOs). There are more than 1000 private insurance companies in the U.S. The benefits, premium, and provider reimbursement methods differ among private insurance plans, as they do in public plans. Physicians, providing both ambulatory and inpatient care are usually paid on a fee-for-service basis with payment rates varying among insurers. Hospitals are reimbursed on the basis of charges, costs, diagnosis-related groups, or negotiated rates, depending on the patient's insurer (Schieber et al., 1992). Costs to third party payers have been reduced by the modern payment method of diagnosis-related groups (DRGs). When a patient enters the hospital, the amount that the hospital will be reimbursed depends on the prospectively determined amount that proper treatment of that condition should cost.

3. Non-patient Revenue and Philanthropy are revenues received for no direct patient care services. Philanthropy is the most recognized source. Philanthropic support may be direct from individuals or from philanthropic organizations such as The United Way.

4. Medicare, enacted in 1965 as Title XVIII of the Social Security Act, is provided to individuals eligible for Social Security and others with chronic disabilities plus voluntary enrollees aged 65 years or more. Effective July 1, 1986, the program provides almost universal health insurance coverage for individuals 65 years and older. In 1987, Medicare covered 45% of all health care expenditures for the elderly (Lazenby et al., 1992). Medicare's role primarily involves financing of acute care services. About 75% of aged Medicare

beneficiaries have some type of private health insurance to defray medical expenses not covered by Medicare, called Medigap policies. Medigap policies are designed to supplement Medicare coverage. Beginning July 30, 1993, 10 standardized insurance policies may be sold to Medicare beneficiaries (Grimaldi, 1992).

5) Medicaid was enacted in 1965 under Title XIX of the Social Security Act. Medicaid is actually a collection of 50 semiautonomous state programs. The programs are jointly financed by state and federal governments, with the Medicaid statute allowing federal outlays from 50-83% of costs incurred depending on the state's economic conditions. In 1987, Mississippi Medicaid program had the largest proportion of federal participation, with the federal government's share at 78.42%. Each state has the responsibility for managing its own program with federal guidelines of established eligibility and range of benefits. Medicaid requires each state to pay for lab and physician fees, x-rays, home health and skilled care, in addition to inpatient and outpatient hospitalization. Each state is required to cover skilled nursing home care, while intermediate care coverage is optional (Buchanan, 1987). Most Medicaid enrollees are young women and children eligible through the Aid to Families with Dependent Children (AFDC) category (Congressional Research Service, 1988). Obstetrical care accounts for a large proportion (33-41%) of Medicaid/AFDC expenditures (Howell & Brown, 1989).

There are no global budget or expenditure limits of health care funding in the U.S. As a result, U.S. healthcare spending is the highest in the world. The health to Gross Domestic Product (GDP) ratio increased from 9.2% in 1980 to 12.1% in 1990, a 2.7% annual rate of growth (Schieber et al., 1992). This high rate of growth is problematic because substantial amounts of non-health sector consumption and investment opportunities are not possible because of the high rate of growth in U.S. health spending (Schieber et al., 1992).

There is currently a tremendous amount of discussion and debate about the monetary allocations for health care. In fact, one of the major issues of the 1992 Presidential campaign between George Bush and Bill Clinton was health care. The major proposals for health care policy were a government run "single payer" system (similar to Canada) and the "play or pay" option which would require employers to provide health insurance for every worker or pay a payroll tax into a government insurance program. Advocates claim the programs will not be expensive because there will be significant savings through cost containment (Hasson, 1992). However, limiting costs to a given percentage of GNP increases the likelihood of rationed health care. After almost three decades of socializing to the entitlements and rights provided by Medicare and Medicaid, Americans may not want to impose a ceiling on health care spending, or they may be unwilling to acquiesce to rationing practices that would ensue (Aaron & Schwartz, 1984).

As health care costs in the U.S. have increased, cost effective measures have become increasingly important in health care delivery. As a result, emergency centers, free-standing clinics, hospital outpatient centers, health maintenance organizations (HMOs) and preferred provider organizations (PPOs) have grown rapidly (Public Health Service, 1988). In addition, the Primary Health Care Model (PHC) is being promoted by many groups (e.g., the World Health Organization) as a global initiative that recognizes the individual as a responsible participant in health care activities (Public Health Service, 1985).

HEALTHY PEOPLE 2000

By the late 1970s, the influence of lifestyle and environmental factors on health promotion and disease prevention had gained national recognition. In 1979, the Public Health Service (PHS) published five major goals for 1990 to reduce premature mortality and morbidity for infants, children, adolescents, youth, adults, and older Americans (PHS, 1979a). The number of health objectives was expanded to 226 in 1980 and expressed as quantitative measures (PHS, 1979b). States and communities identified priority areas and developed programs for disease prevention and health promotion. Also, private businesses, voluntary agencies, schools, hospitals, and federal agencies instituted plans. As a result, progress toward meeting the objectives was reported in 1986 for a midcourse review, documenting that 13% of the 226 objectives had been achieved and should be obtained by 1990, and 26% had no data to measure progress (McFarlane, 1989; PHS, 1986).

In September 1990, *Healthy People 2000: National Health Promotion and Disease Prevention Objectives* were unveiled. The year 2000 initiative is the result of three years of formulation with the comments of more than 10,000 people including national, state, and local agencies and communities, private and voluntary groups, consumers, and other individuals. The Healthy People 2000 initiative emphasizes the full range of functional capacity from infancy to old age and includes measures of health outcomes (Public Health Service, 1991a).

WOMEN'S HEALTH IN THE UNITED STATES

Most health care is provided by women, either as informal caregivers in their roles as mothers, grandmothers, wives, daughters of the elderly, or as neighbors (World Health Organization, 1983). Women shape their own health and the health of their families through their individual concepts of health and illness (Lempert, 1986). In the formal health sector, women are the majority of practitioners. However, the health needs of women are frequently neglected, their contributions to health development undervalued, and their working conditions ignored (World Health Organization, 1983).

Child Care

In 1988, 68% of U.S. children 5 years or younger had been in a child care arrangement at some time in their lives (56% less than 2 years; 80% 4-5 years who were not in school). Whether a child receives care outside of the home is strongly associated with the socioeconomic status of the household, with 79% of children from families earning greater than $40,000 and 48% of children from families earning less than $10,000 annually. Nearly all (98%) of children in child care had mothers' who worked. Moreover, the percentage of children ever cared for in regular arrangements increased with the mother's education attainment: 78% of children in arranged child care had mothers who had attended college. One-third of children whose mothers did not work had been in some child care arrangement during their lives (Dawson, 1990). The main sources of arranged care were nursery or preschool (23%), nonrelative in a home other than the child's own home (21%), child's fathe (13%), in child's home by related providers (8%), and in child's home by ul related providers (6%) (Dawson, 1990).

Cancer and Cancer Prevention

Breast cancer is the leading cause of cancer deaths in females. It is the second most common cause of cancer deaths behind lung cancer. However, in women, the incidence of breast cancer is two times that of lung cancer. In 1990, an estimated 150,000 new cases of breast cancer were diagnosed (Public Health Service, 1991b). During the remainder of the decade, more than 1.5 million women will be diagnosed with breast cancer and nearly 30% will die. Clinical breast exams and mammography can detect lesions at a curable stage in women (National Institutes of Health, 1991). In 1990, about 47% of women aged 50 years or more had received a clinical breast exam and a mammogram within the last two years (Public Health Service, 1991b).

Weinberger et al. (1991) found that physicians screen elderly women (75+ years) less often than younger women. They speculated that reduced screening of older women may be the result of age-bias or confusion about the appropriate screening intervals for this age group. Also, their study found that the cost of mammography was a barrier for all age groups.

Since 1969, there has been a decrease of 50% in deaths from cervical cancer. In 1989, there were 4,487 women who died from cervical cancer. In 1990, 93% of all women age 18 or older had reported having a Papanicolaou (Pap) test, with about 81% within the last 3 years. This figure represents the greatest proportion of adults screened for any type of cancer. About 77% of Hispanic women, 69% of women ages 70 and over, 70% of women who did not finish high school, and 72% of women with low family incomes had a Pap test within 3 years (Public Health Service, 1991b).

In 1989, 63% of Medicaid recipients were women. Of those, 64% were aged 15-84 years, corresponding to guidelines for Pap smear screening, and 22% were between 45-84 years, ages appropriate for mammography. Twenty-six states provide coverage of Pap exams for all eligible women covered. Ten states cover the costs with an M.D. order, five states cover only lab costs, and seven states cover women eligible to be seen in family planning or maternity clinics. Two states, Georgia and Nevada provide no coverage for Pap tests. It is estimated that there are 680,000 Medicaid women eligible for Pap exams for whom partial payment is not provided. Twenty-three states provide coverage of mammography for eligible women, and 16 cover the costs if there is an M.D. order. Twelve states provide no coverage for eligible women, or 570,000 Medicaid-eligible women for whom there is no coverage (Boss & Guckes, 1992).

AIDS and AIDS Prevention

Between January 1987 and November 1991 the number of AIDS cases among women in the U.S. increased by over 1,000% to 20,739 cases. In the U.S., women represent 10% of all AIDS cases. The majority of women with AIDS (72%) are black or Hispanic, poor, and disadvantaged. The total number of AIDS cases among women in December 1990 was equal to the total number of AIDS cases among men 5 years earlier. The primary route of infection for women is about 51% from injected drugs, while 32% acquire the disease from heterosexual contact. Human immunodeficiency virus (HIV) exposure through heterosexual contact differs greatly between men and women with 32% of female AIDS cases resulting through contact, while 2% of men had (Ickovics & Rodin, 1992).

High risk women for HIV exposure include sex partners of injectable drug users, black and Hispanic women, prostitutes, and adolescents. However, it is important to emphasize that it is lack of preventive behaviors, not membership in a particular group, that exposes a woman to HIV infection. Nearly two-thirds (63%) of women with AIDS who contracted the disease through heterosexual contact were sex partners of men who used intravenous drugs; and they had no history of drug use themselves. Black and Hispanic women are 11 times more likely to acquire HIV infection through heterosexual contact because of the traditional lack of barrier contraceptive use and the ethnic, cultural, and religious influences surrounding sexual behavior and condom use (Ickovics & Rodin, 1992).

Professional sex workers have higher HIV risks because of multiple sex partners, high-risk sexual activity (e.g., anal sex), IV drug use, and reduced vigilance about safe-sex practices. Adolescents are categorized as high-risk because of sexual and drug experimentation, the tendency to engage in high-risk behavior, a sense of invulnerability and immortality, less well-developed coping styles and cognitive processing, and reduced access to age-appropriate social and medical services (Ickovics & Rodin, 1992).

AIDS brings forth the significant issue of health-promoting behavior and how to address ethnic differences between white, black, and Hispanic populations when attempting to disseminate information. The groups require culturally and linguistically appropriate information for the different age groups.

Abortion and Family Planning

In 1989, there were 34.6 therapeutic abortions per 1000 women, an increase from 27.1 in 1987. The majority of abortions were performed on unmarried women, with a rate of 88.4 per 1000. The rate for married women in 1989 was 7.8 per 1000. There were ethnic differences among women who had abortions, with 24.8 per 1000 among white women and 46.1 for blacks and others. Interestingly, the rate of abortions among white women has increased from 22.6 per 1000 in 1985 and decreased in black women to 55.5 per 1000 the same year.

Abortion services are heavily concentrated in urban areas, with 25% of all abortions performed in five metropolitan areas. Only 14% of women of reproductive age live in these areas, New York, Los Angeles, Chicago, the District of Columbia, and San Francisco. There are 70 of 305 metropolitan areas that have no abortion providers. There are 12 million women in rural areas and 2.5 million women in the 70 smaller cities who would have difficulties obtaining abortion services. All regions of the country and one-half of all states have metropolitan areas with no providers. Indiana, Ohio, Pennsylvania, Texas, and Wisconsin each have five or more metropolitan areas without abortion services (Updates, 1992).

In the U.S. the risk of death from childbearing for teens is 14 times higher than from an abortion. Twenty-eight percent of teenagers (12-17 years) have had sexual intercourse and many do not use birth control. Sexual activity begins earlier among teens who have the fewest resources (WIPHN News, 1989).

Women and Aging

Aging is a special concern for women, because women live longer than men. The population of the U.S. is getting older. From 1980-1990, the population aged 85 years and over grew by 3.8% annually compared with 202% for those aged 65+ and 4.6% for those 35-44 years. While the oldest old (85+ years) represent a small percent of the population, they are a growing group. Individuals, families, and governments have begun planning for their well-being, but significant health, social, and economic needs of the elderly are currently unmet.

Elderly women outnumber elderly men 3 to 2, and the disparity grows larger in the upper age ranges. In 1989, there were 84 men for every 100 women between the ages of 65 and 69. Among the 85+ population, there were only 39 men for every 100 women. Therefore, elderly women are more likely than men to end up living alone. The 1990 census counted 35,808 centenarians, or nearly

12 of every 10,000 elderly persons aged 65+. About 78.5% of centenarians are women. Nearly one-half of women aged 60 can expect to reach at least 85; for men the probability is 1 in 4 (Suzman, Manton, & Willis, 1992).

In addition to sex differences in longevity, there are ethnic differences. In 1989, 13% of whites were 65+, compared with 8% of blacks, 7% of other ethnic origins (Native Americans and Asian/Pacific Islanders), and 5% of Hispanics. However, the older minority population is expected to increase in the next century because of the higher fertility rate of nonwhite and Hispanic populations (U.S. Senate Committee on Aging, 1991).

Women are more likely than men to live in institutional settings, 26.3% versus 16.1% (Schneider & Guralnik, 1990). In 1980, about 509,000 (22%) of the population 85+ lived in institutionalized settings, which included homes for the aged (488,000; 92%), mental institutions (7,000; 1%), and others, i.e., homes for handicapped (14,000; 3%).

In the U.S., 6% of women and 3% of men live in nursing homes (Schneider & Guralnik, 1990). There are two major classes of nursing homes, skilled and intermediate. Skilled nursing homes (SNH) provide 24-hour nursing services, regular medical supervision, and daily rehabilitation therapy on an inpatient basis. They must meet established laws and regulations of health and safety. Intermediate care facilities are also called health-related facilities (HRF). They are licensed under a state law to provide health-related care and services on a regular basis to persons who do not require the degree of care and treatment provided by a hospital or skilled nursing facility (Brickner, Lechich, Lipsman, & Scharer, 1987).

For particular age groups, the nursing home population increases from 1% of men and women aged 65-74 years to 15% of men and 25% of women 85+ years. Only 4% of women in nursing homes were married compared to 23% of men. Three of five men in nursing homes had less than 8 years of education, while one-half of women did; 28% of men and 36% of women in nursing homes were at least high school graduates (Schneider & Guralnik, 1990).

The percentage of women who live at home and need the help of someone else increases from 10% of those 65-74 years to 37% for those 85+. For men, 9% between the ages of 65-74 years and 31% of those aged 85+ live at home and need help from someone else. Therefore, the majority of women (62%) and a significant number of men (46%) aged 85+ years either live in nursing homes or need assistance to live at home. Forty-five percent of elderly nursing home residents are 85+ years of age (Schneider & Guralnik, 1990).

American Women and Violence

The crime rate against women in the U.S. is significantly higher than in other countries. The U.S. has a rape rate that is 13 times higher than England, 4 times greater than Germany and 20 times higher than Japan (Taeuber, 1991).

Up to one-third of women treated in the emergency rooms of U.S. hospitals have been abused (Headlines, 1992). One-third of all domestic violence, if reported, would be charged as a felony, rape, or felonious assault. Approximately 50% of all rapes are reported, with less than 40% resulting in arrests. In addition, a woman is battered every 15 seconds and 8% of pregnant women are abused. Not only are young women battered, but elderly women are as well. There are reportedly 700,000-1,300,000 reports of elder abuse each year (Meierhoffer, 1992). This is a significant women's health concern as older women significantly outnumber older men, especially those 85+ years.

Health care delivery in the U.S. has become a site of violence in some areas. Nurses in hospital emergency rooms and psychiatric facilities are at greatest risk. One study reported that of 1200 emergency room RN respondents, 97% had experienced some type of victimization (violence, threat of violence, intimidation, extortion, theft of property, etc.). Verbal abuse was most common, followed by threats and intimidation and physical assault. Most victimizers were patients (Selby, 1992). Selby also reported that one study showed 36% of nurses had been physically assaulted within the previous 12 months.

The University of Alabama at Birmingham installed a metal detector at the entrance to the ambulatory and emergency services in October 1991. More than 500 weapons, from handguns to icepicks, have been confiscated (Selby, 1992).

SUMMARY

The U.S. health care system has begun to focus on prevention and education instead of diagnosis and treatment. Given the diversity of the U.S., no one health care plan can effectively care for all Americans. While the majority of Americans are white, there are many other ethnic groups, with different health care practices that are not recognized by traditional Western medicine. Each ethnic group should be given the opportunity to maintain health practices within the U.S. system as health and illness are defined and described in cultural terms. In particular, women should become the focus of health care as they are the cornerstone of all health care.

Community-based health care is culturally sensitive and geographically accessible. American communities are ethnically diverse. Each community should be responsible for determining appropriate health care issues that need to be addressed by their particular population. The issues should be determined not only by health care providers but also by community members not affiliated with health organizations. Only by recognizing the vast differences within the population will effective policies be made.

The ability of nurses to contain health costs, particularly in nursing centers, long-term and home care, plus the public trust of nurses, demonstrates the important role nurses will play in reforming health care (National League for

Nursing, 1990). The Primary Health Care Model deserves greater attention in future health care reforms because it emphasizes prevention and individual and community responsibility for health preservation and the prevention of disease and illness. A focus on prevention and education, not diagnosis and cure, can make a major contribution to better and less costly health care for women and for all Americans.

REFERENCES

Aaron, H. J., & Schwartz, W. B. (1984). *The painful prescription: Rationing hospital care*. Washington, DC: Brookings Institution.

Boss, L. P., & Guckes, F. H. (1992). Medicaid coverage of screening tests for breast and cervical cancer. *American Journal of Public Health, 82*(2), 252-253.

Brickner, P.W., Lechich, A. J., Lipsman, R., & Scharer, L. K. (1987). *Long-term health care*. New York: Basic Books, Inc.

Buchanan, R. J. (1987). *Medicaid: Cost containment*. Cranberry, NJ: Association of University Presses, Inc.

Bureau of Health Professions. (1990). *1988 Sample survey of registered nurses*. Division of Nursing. Washington, DC.

Congressional Research Service. (1988). *Medicaid source book: Background data and analysis*. Washington, DC: United States Government Printing Office.

Data Watch. (1991). More households give to health care organizations. *Hospitals, 65*(8), 16.

Dawson, D. A. (1990). Child care arrangements: Health of our nation's children, United States, 1988. *Advance Data from Vital and Health Statistics*. No. 187. National Center for Health Sciences.

Grimaldi, P. (1992). Medigap insurance policies standardized. *Nursing Management, 23*(11), 20.

Hasson, J. (1992, October 15). No simple cure for sick system. *USA Today*, p. 5A.

Headlines. (1992). *American Journal of Nursing, 92*(3), 9.

Howell, E. M., & Brown, G. A. (1989). Prenatal, delivery and infant care under Medicaid in three states. *Health Care Financing Review, 10*, 1-15.

Ickovics, J. R. (1992). Epidemiology of women and AIDS in the United States. *Women's Health Forum, 1*(4), 1-2.

Lazenby, H. C., Levit, K. R., Waldo, D. R., Adler, G. S., Letsch, S. W. & Cowan, C. A. (1992). National health accounts: Lessons from the U.S. experience. *Health Care Financing Review, 13*(4), 89-104.

Lempert, L. B. (1986). Women's health from a woman's point of view: A review of the literature. *Health Care for Women International, 7*, 255-275.

McFarlane, J. (1989). Year 2000 health objectives for the nation. *Public Health Nursing, 6*(2), 51-54.

Meierhoffer, L. L. (1992). Nurses battle family violence. *The American Nurse, 24*(4), 1.

National Institutes of Health. (1990). *Consensus statement: Early stage breast cancer. 8*(6), 2-3.

National League for Nursing. (1990). *Nationwide survey of attitudes toward health care and nurses.* New York: Peter D. Hart Research Associates.

National League for Nursing. (1992). *Nursing data review 1992,* New York.

Pink, L. A. (1991). Hospitals. In J. E. Finchham and A. I. Wertheimer (Eds.). *Pharmacy and the U.S. health care system,* New York:Pharmaceutical Products Press.

Public Health Service. (1979a). *Healthy people: The Surgeon General's report on health promotion and disease: Prevention.* Washington, DC: United States Government Printing Office.

Public Health Service (1979b). *Healthy people: The Surgeon General's report on health promotion and disease prevention: Background papers.* Washington, DC: United States Government Printing Office.

Public Health Service. (1985). *Women's health.* Report of the Public Health Service Task Force on Women's Health Issues (Vol. II). Washington, DC: United States Department of Health and Human Services.

Public Health Service. (1986). *The 1990 health objectives for the nation: A midcourse review.* Washington, DC: United States Government Printing Office.

Public Health Service. (1988). *Nursing: Sixth report to the President and Congress on the status of health personnel in the United States.* Washington, DC: United States Department of Health and Human Services.

Public Health Service. (1991). *Health United States: 1990.* (DHHS Publication No. (PHS) 91-1232). Hyattsville, MA: National Center for Health Statistics.

Public Health Service. (1991). *Healthy people 2000: National health promotion and disease prevention objectives.* (DHHS Pub. No. (PHS) 91-50213)

Roemer, M. I. (1991). Entrepreneurial health systems in industrialized countries. In M. I. Roemer (Ed.), *National health systems of the world, Vol. I: The countries.* New York: Oxford University Press.

Schieber, G. J., Poullier, J., & Greenwald, L. M. (1992). U.S. health expenditure performance: An international comparison and data update. *Health Care Financing Review, 13*(4), 1-13.

Schneider, E. L., & Guralnik, J. M. (1990). The aging of America: Impact on health care costs. *Journal of the American Medical Association, 263*(17), 2335-2340.

Selby, T. L. (1992). Nurses face growing risk of violence and abuse. *The American Nurse, 24*(4), 3.

Sidel, R. (1992). Women and children first: Towards a U.S. family policy. *American Journal of Public Health*, *82*(5), 664-665.

Special Report. (1992). Wasted health care dollars. *Consumer Reports*, *57*(7), 435-448.

Suzman, R. M., Manton, K. G., & Willis, D. P. (1992). *The oldest old*. New York: Oxford University Press.

Taeuber, C. (1991). *Statistical handbook on women in America*. Phoenix, AZ: Oryx Press.

U.S. Senate Special Committee on Aging. (1991). *Aging America: Trends and projections*.

Updates. (1992). *Health Care Financing Review*, *13*(4), 205.

Weinburger, M., Saunders, A. F., Samsa, G. P., Bearon, L. B., Gold, D. T., Brown, J. T., Booher, P., & Loehrer, P. J. (1991). Breast cancer screening in older women: Practices and barriers reported by primary care physicians. *Journal of the American Geriatric Society*, *39*(22), 22-27.

WIPHN News. (1989). *Women's International Public Health Network*, *6*, 1.

World Health Organization. (1983). Women as providers of health care. *WHO Chronicle*, *37*(4), 134-138.

8

Women's Health Status in the United States: A Chicago Perspective

Collaborating Center for International Nursing Development
in Primary Health Care
The University of Illinois at Chicago
College of Nursing

Beverly J. McElmurry

INTRODUCTION

The United States of America (USA) is a federal republic of 50 states. In 1988, there were 243,915,000 people, 51% of whom were women (U.S. Department of Commerce, Bureau of Census, 1989). The majority (83.1%) of the population are white, 11.6% are black, 6.5% are of Spanish origin, and the remainder are Native American Indians and Asian. English is the predominant language, but a sizable minority speaks Spanish (Table 8-1).

Health care in the United States is delivered via dual, public/private systems. Health care is delivered primarily on a fee-for-service basis by a variety of practitioners. Until relatively recently, hospitals were the major sites of health care delivery in the U.S. However, a number of alternative modes of health care delivery have proliferated in recent years. The importance of providing care in the most cost-effective settings has resulted in rapid increases in the number of free standing clinics, emergency centers, and hospital outpatient centers. Health

Table 8-1. Country Demographics: United States of America

WHO Region	Americas
Size	9,363,353 square kilometers
Land use	32% forest, 29% grazing, 19% cultivated, 22% waste, urban, other
Climate	Temperate and semi-arid
Government	Federated republic
Total population	244 million (1988)
Female population	51.3%
Annual growth rate	0.9%
Religion	Protestant, Roman Catholic
Language	English
Capital	Washington, DC
Rural/Urban	Mixed
Main export	Agriculture, industry
Literacy rate	99% women, 99% men
Life expectancy	78 women, 70 men

Maintenance Organizations (HMOs) and Preferred Provider Organizations (PPOs) have grown rapidly (Public Health Service, 1988, p. vii). Numbers of health care personnel have increased in most parts of the country. In general, this increase has exceeded the growth rate of the population. However, many geographic areas still lack sufficient numbers of practitioners to assure adequate access to care. It is estimated that about 13 million persons (5%) of the United States population are underserved (Public Health Service, 1988, p. vi). Financial access to health care is also a major concern in the U.S. Although third party payment is available for much of the population, some segments of the population, of which women are a growing proportion, do not have financial access to care.

In addition to changes in the methods of payment and delivery of health care, fundamental changes are occurring in the way the nation's health problems are viewed. It is now recognized that technological "breakthroughs" are unlikely to continue to contribute substantially to improvements in health status. Rather, the emphasis is beginning to shift to environment and social changes, changes in lifestyle, and participation of people in maintaining and promoting their own health (Public Health Service, 1988, p. I-1). Causes of mortality and morbidity have shifted from infectious disease to chronic illness and accidents. Therefore, the need to focus on health policies that promote healthy conditions and behaviors has received increasing attention in the United States (Public Health Service, 1985, p. I-1).

In an effort to respond to the mandate for health for all by the year 2000, the United States, under Title XVII of the Public Health Services Act, directed the

Secretary of Health and Human Services to establish national preventive health goals (McFarlane, 1989). In Tables 8-2 and 8-3, selected data are presented about U.S. women that will influence health promotion goals and activities.

Women and Primary Health Care

At the end of the United Nations Decade for Women, the World Health Organization (WHO) prepared a report on and proposed primary health care (PHC) strategies regarding women's health (1985). PHC is promoted as a global initiative which recognizes the individual as a responsible participant in health care activities. The report suggested "that messages meant to be received by women [be] relevant to their health priorities and...suitably presented...[and] that

Table 8-2. Social and Economic Profile of US Women

Births
- In 1988, there were 66 births per 1000 white women, 87 for black women and 94 for Hispanic women between 18 to 44 years
- Childbearing has increased among women over age 30 and under age 16
- By 1987, women had fewer than two children each, and birthrates for white, black and Hispanics will continue to drop in the 1990s
- Babies are born out of wedlock in 3 of 4 black births, 2 of 10 white births, and 3 of 10 Hispanic births
- Teenagers and women over 40 are the most likely to have an abortion

Women and Work
- Fifty-seven (57) percent of all women were in the labor force in 1989
- Over half of women with infants are in the labor force
- Employers have work-schedule policies that aid child care more than providing benefits or services
- The majority of women are still in traditional low-paying "female" occupations and earn less than men with the same education
- Few women are self-employed or owners of American firms

Women and Poverty
- More than one in three women who maintain families work full time but earn less than poverty level income
- The relative economic disadvantage of families maintained by women alone appears to be growing
- Only half of the women awarded child support received the amount awarded and most poor women are not awarded child support
- Four out of five long-term unmarried mothers receive welfare
- One in five mothers with a child under age three was poor
- The majority of poor women are high school dropouts

Source: Taeuber (1991).

Table 8-3. Health Profile of US Women

Health and Illness[a]
- Like men, roughly one in 20 women has a work disability
- Flu and the common cold are the most frequently occurring conditions for women
- Arthritis is a major chronic condition for women
- Cancer of the breast occurs more than any other type among women, and the incidence of lung cancer has increased in women
- Very few women are heavy drinkers
- Most women aged 18 to 34 have used illegal drugs at some time
- Anti-infectives are the most frequently prescribed drugs for women

Women and AIDS[b]
- AIDS Diagnosis—13,395 women by 1990
- Source of Infections:
  - 51%—IV drug use
  - 32%—Heterosexual contact
  - 10%—Blood transfusion
  - 7%—Undetermined
- 72% of total women with AIDS are black or Hispanic

Death and Aging[a]
- Death rates for American children, especially teenagers, are generally higher than in most developed countries
- Women, like men, are most likely to die of heart disease and cancer
- American teenage girls are much more likely to be murdered than are teenage girls in other countries
- The number of women 65 years and over will at least double in the next 10 years
- Many elderly women have trouble with heavy housework, shopping and walking
- White women 85 years and over are the most likely to be residents of a nursing home

[a]*Source:* Taeuber (1991).

[b]*Source:* Watstein & Laurich (1991).

women have access to appropriate health education that will enable them to better play their role as health providers, particularly at the family level" (p. 24).

Among the strategies proposed specifically by the WHO for the Region of the Americas (Pan American Health Organization—PAHO) are the following:
1. "promote research and collection and analysis of data in order to define and identify relevant problems and issues" (p. 32), and

2. "ensure that women are involved and that their needs are taken into account in development projects and activities in primary health care" (p. 33).

The World Federation of Public Health Associations, in their "Information for Action Issue Paper: Women and Health" (1986), concurred that "problems of older women and men have not been adequately recognized in primary health care" (p. 17).

The College of Nursing as a designated WHO Collaborating Centre for Primary Health Care and as the Secretariat for a global network of nursing collaborating centres is in an important position for contributing to the PHC of women. The College of Nursing has made commitments to meet WHO priorities; to promote PHC and HFA 2000; to emphasize cross-cultural understanding of women's health concerns in our administrative, research, and teaching activities; and to promote international collaboration in nursing research, education, and policy recommendations.

Educating and caring for women helps them take better care of themselves, their families, and communities. WHO (1983) enumerated eight ways in which women provide primary health care:

1. educating family members to promote health and prevent disease,
2. processing, storing, and preparing food supplies and ensuring proper nutrition,
3. hauling, storing, and distributing water and managing basic sanitation for the family and often also for the community,
4. immunizing themselves and their children,
5. providing maternal and child care; initiating self-help; and deciding if and when family members will utilize health services,
6. preventing, controlling, diagnosing, and treating locally prevalent diseases,
7. treating common diseases and injuries in the home and giving first aid,
8. producing and collecting the basic ingredients of some drugs, and keeping drugs away from dampness and heat and out of reach of children. (pp. 134-138)

UIC Women's Health Concentration

Since 1977, the College of Nursing has housed a group of faculty and a steady stream of students from many countries who share a strong interest in research, teaching, and practice related to women's health. As a consequence of this interest, the Graduate Nursing Concentration in Women's Health was added to the College of Nursing curriculum in 1984 to encourage students to study and conduct research on primary health care, self care, minority health, and international health issues (Figure 8-1). The Women's Health Concentration has facilitated the development of an international cadre of nurses with expertise in

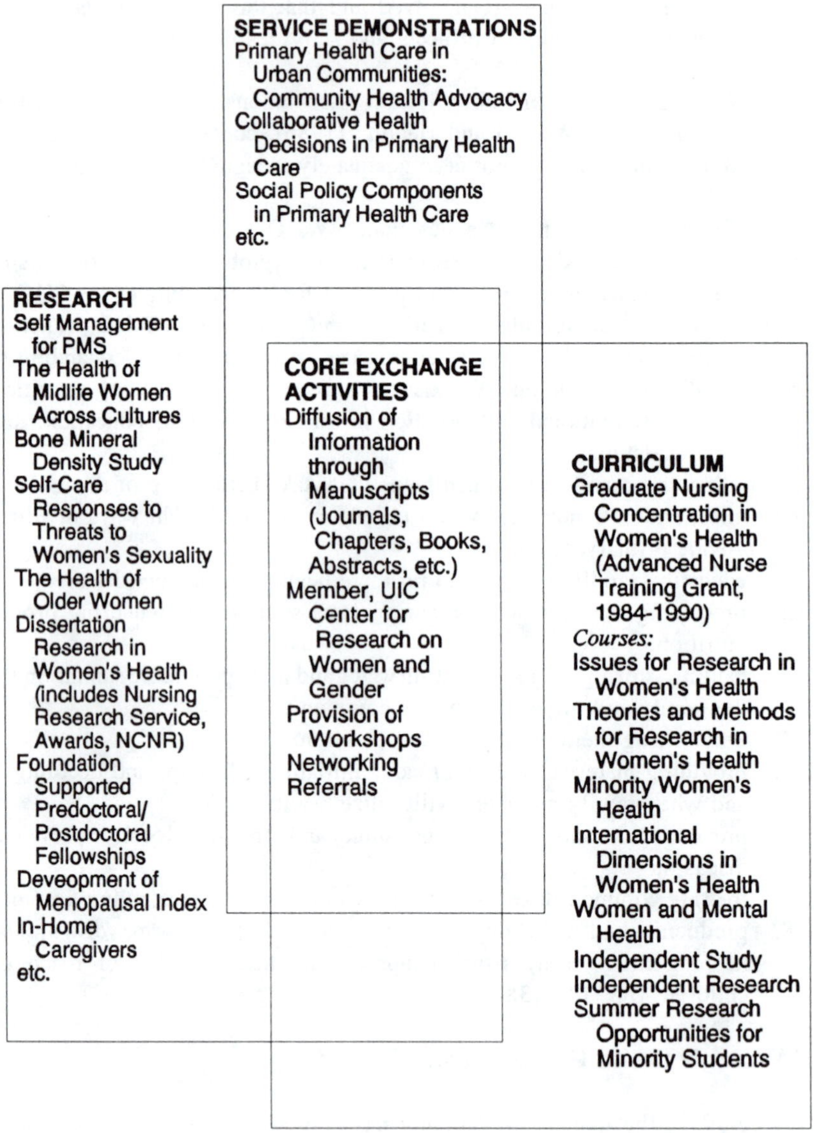

SERVICE DEMONSTRATIONS
Primary Health Care in
  Urban Communities:
  Community Health Advocacy
Collaborative Health
  Decisions in Primary Health
  Care
Social Policy Components
  in Primary Health Care
etc.

RESEARCH
Self Management
  for PMS
The Health of
  Midlife Women
  Across Cultures
Bone Mineral
  Density Study
Self-Care
  Responses to
  Threats to
  Women's Sexuality
The Health of
  Older Women
Dissertation
  Research in
  Women's Health
  (includes Nursing
  Research Service,
  Awards, NCNR)
Foundation
  Supported
  Predoctoral/
  Postdoctoral
  Fellowships
Deveopment of
  Menopausal Index
In-Home
  Caregivers
etc.

**CORE EXCHANGE
ACTIVITIES**
Diffusion of
  Information
  through
  Manuscripts
  (Journals,
  Chapters, Books,
  Abstracts, etc.)
Member, UIC
  Center for
  Research on
  Women and
  Gender
Provision of
  Workshops
Networking
Referrals

CURRICULUM
Graduate Nursing
  Concentration in
  Women's Health
  (Advanced Nurse
  Training Grant,
  1984-1990)
Courses:
Issues for Research in
  Women's Health
Theories and Methods
  for Research in
  Women's Health
Minority Women's
  Health
International
  Dimensions in
  Women's Health
Women and Mental
  Health
Independent Study
Independent Research
Summer Research
  Opportunities for
  Minority Students

Figure 8-4. Women's Health Program, The University of Illinois at Chicago, College of Nursing.

women's health. The Women's Health Exchange, based in the College of Nursing, serves as a resource and information center for consumers and providers as well as local, regional, national, and international scholars and organizations which share an interest in women's health. As a result of the research done by its faculty and students, the College of Nursing and the Women's Health Exchange have an expanding database of information on women's health in many countries.

The UIC program holds the following assumptions about the health care of women:

- The human body, mind, and spirit form a whole.
- Women have the capacity for self-care and self-healing.
- Events and interactions in the family, community, and world affect and shape the health of women.
- Health care is a shared responsibility.
- Health reflects integrity, flexibility, capacity to develop, and capacity to creatively transcend difficult situations.
- Control over one's body is a basic right.
- Lived experiences are the starting point for future action.
- Women's health settings vary.
- The health of all is improved by focusing on women's health. (McElmurry & Huddleston, 1991)

In Fall 1991, the UIC Campus Center for Research on Women and Gender (CRWG) opened after 5 years of planning. As a campus-wide Center with some state funding support, the Center staff are expected to obtain grants and contracts to advance interdisciplinary research on women's health.

The purpose of the CRWG is to promote collaborative, multidisciplinary research related to women and gender, particularly in the areas of culture, work, and health. By bringing together a cadre of outstanding UIC scholars, the Center can advance the collaboration necessary to address serious gender-related issues facing society today.

The goals of the Center are to:

- Stimulate and increase knowledge about women and about gender as an explanatory category of research,
- Study and evaluate the impact of policies related to women and gender,
- Increase the dissemination and use of new scholarship on women and gender, and
- Create alliances with outside organizations sharing interests in women and gender-related issues.

The Center will be a resource for efforts to improve the climate for women faculty and students. In addition, it is a focus and mechanism for drawing funding to research on women and gender from both government and private sources.

Among the Center's current and planned activities are the following:

- Women's Health Research: Strategies and Opportunities for Change—a conference for specialists in women's health, cosponsored with the Society for the Advancement of Women's Health Research.
- National Conference on Multidisciplinary Specialization in Women's Health.
- Changing Women/Changing Science—a conference to improve access to careers in science and engineering for women.
- Agents of Continuity and Change: Mexican, Chicana, and Indian Women—a conference cosponsored with the UIC Latin American Studies program.
- Campus support group at the University of Illinois at Chicago for women graduate students in science.
- An on-line directory of faculty interested in issues related to women and gender.
- Visiting scholars program.

The recently released *Findings of the 1991 Women's Health Research Roundtables* emphasize that a women's health research agenda is a metaphor or symbol for the conceptual and systematic changes that are needed to act collectively to improve the health of women. The two day roundtables represented invited groups of providers and consumers and were held in three USA locations (Albuquerque, New Mexico; Raleigh, North Carolina; and Chicago, Illinois). The Chicago roundtable was cosponsored by the UIC CRWG. The roundtables identified themes that are characteristic of a biopsychosocial approach to understanding health. The emerging themes indicate the importance of attending to:

- Self-Esteem and Women's Health
- Mental Health and Substance Abuse
- Causes of and Treatment for AIDS/Immunological Diseases
- Teenage Pregnancy
- Contraceptive Research

In addition to the themes which emerged from the conference, attention was paid to the conceptual and systemic changes needed in women's health. These concerns included recognizing the adversity of women; the importance of aggressive attention to the prevention of illness as well as intervention to cure illness; finding ways to bridge the Biomedical/Psychosocial dichotomy; attending to the many methodological issues in the conduct of women's health research; and finding means to adequately fund women's health research, including community-based participants. It was also recognized that research must help us achieve access to health care and deal with some of the provider issues in health care for women.

REFERENCES

McElmurry, B. J., & Huddleston, D. S. (1991). Self-Care and menopause: Critical review of research. *Health Care for Women International, 12*, 15-26.

McFarlane, J. (1989). Year 2000 health objectives for the nation. *Public Health Nursing, 6*(2), 51-54.

Public Health Service (1985). *Women's health*. Report of the Public Health Service Task Force on Women's Health Issues (Vol. II). Washington, DC: United States Department of Health and Human Services.

Public Health Service (1988). *Nursing: Sixth report to the President and Congress on the status of health personnel in the United States*. Washington, DC: United States Department of Health and Human Services.

Society for the Advancement of Women's Health Research (1992). *Findings of the 1991 Women's Health Research Roundtables*. Washington, DC.

Taeuber, C. (1991). *Statistical handbook on women in America*. Phoenix, AZ: Oryx Press.

U.S. Department of Commerce (1989). *Statistical abstract of the United States* (109th ed.) Washington, DC: Bureau of Census.

Watstein, S. B., & Laurich, R. A. (1991). *AIDS and women: A sourcebook*. Phoenix, AZ: Oryx Press.

WHO (1983). Women as providers of health care. *WHO Chronicle, 37*(4), 134-138.

World Federation of Public Health Associations (1986, March). *Women and health: Information for Action Issue Paper*. Geneva: World Federation of Public Health Associations.

World Health Organization. (1985). *Women, health and development* (Publication No. 90). Geneva, Switzerland: World Health Organization.

9

Women's Health Status in the United States: Maternal and Child Health

Collaborating Centre for International Nursing Development
in Research, Leadership and Education
University of Pennsylvania
School of Nursing

Health care during pregnancy is a major women's health issue. Adequate prenatal care, including provision for adequate nutrition, can have a major impact on the current and future health of a woman and her infant. Adequate and early prenatal care has been shown to be the single most cost-effective health care strategy for reducing infant mortality in the United States. Normal births account for the largest single category of hospital admissions. The United States has one of the highest per capita health care expenditures in the world, yet our infant mortality ranks only seventeenth. This relatively poor performance reflects a health care system that contains numerous economic, psychological, social, and cultural barriers to prenatal care. These barriers are especially prevalent for poor women and minority women. Lack of adequate prenatal care and prevention not only contributes to high infant mortality but also drives up overall health care costs because so many premature infants require prolonged intensive care.

A brief review of childbearing patterns in the United States, prenatal care received, and maternal and infant birth outcomes highlights the need for improvement in maternal child health in the United States. Current patterns regarding place of birth and care provider are examined. Finally, the nation's goals for maternal child health and current funding initiatives to provide maternal child health services are discussed. Greater national attention to maternal health needs of women will have a major impact on women's overall health, infant mortality, and health care costs.

BIRTHS[6]

In 1989, 4,040,958 babies were born in the United States, with a birth rate of 16.3 and fertility rate of 69.2, an increase of 3% over 1988 for both indicators (1). Approximately 79% of these births were to white women, 17% to black women, and 4.3% to mothers of other races. Birth rates increased for all age specific groups, but the greatest increases were for young teens 15-17 and women 35-44 years of age. These rates increased to the highest level in 15 years.

For young teens the birth rate rose to 36.5 per 1000 births, 8% higher than 1988 and 19% higher than in 1986. This increase reflects social trends to earlier sexual activity for women in the United States, combined with lack of effective contraception among adolescents. Inadequacies in U.S. sex education programs and family planning services contribute to this problem. Early and unprotected intercourse exposes young teens to numerous health and socioeconomic risks, including unwanted motherhood, exposure to sexually transmitted diseases and AIDS, interrupted education, and lower economic opportunity. Minority adolescents suffer disproportionately from the negative consequences of adolescent births. By age 18, black adolescents are four times as likely, and Hispanics twice as likely, as white adolescents, to become mothers (2). Although birth rates for adolescents 16-19 years old have declined steadily over the last 10 years, the United States still has the highest incidence of adolescent childbearing of any industrialized nation.

For women 35-39 there was a 6% increase in the birth rate over 1988 to 29.7; in comparison the rate in 1980 was 19.8. For women 40-44, the birth rate is 5.2 per 1000, an 8% increase over 1988 and 33% higher than in 1980. The rise in rates for women over 35 reflects an increased number of post-World War II baby boomers in this age group as well as their decision to make up for delayed childbearing due to career choices.

Birth rates to unmarried women rose to 41.8 per 1000, 8% higher than in 1988 and 42% higher than in 1980. Birth rates to unmarried women have demonstrated a greater than 5% increase each year over the past 5 years,

---

[6]Unless otherwise noted, all natality and mortality statistics are taken from National Center for Health Statistics Reports, 1991 and 1992.

reflecting a continuing social trend to childbearing outside marriage. This trend, coupled with a continued high divorce rate, has led to an increased number of single woman and their children living in poverty. While many single mothers receive strong support from their family of origin and/or a male partner, others lack adequate social support and a stable male presence in the household. The average income of a single mother family is about 40% of that of two parent families of the same age. Today one out of every five children in the United States lives in a family with income below the poverty level; 44% of black children live in poverty compared with 15% of white children (3).

Adolescent births continue to be a significant problem with over half a million births to adolescent mothers each year. In 1989 the birth rate for adolescents 15-17 years of age was 36.5 per 1000, the highest rate in 15 years and 19% higher than in 1986 (4). The birth rate per 1000 was 49.2 for white mothers under 20 years of age, as compared to 115.4 for black and 103.1 for Hispanics (4). Among unmarried mothers, birth rates continue to be highest for those aged 18-24 years, with rates of 57-62 per 1000 births. While a great deal of attention has been given the unwed teen mother, relatively little attention has been given to the needs of older unmarried mothers, a substantial and increasing group.

PRENATAL CARE

Nowhere is the lack of attention to preventive care in the U.S. health care system more starkly revealed than in the area of prenatal care. Despite spiraling health care costs, the proportion of women receiving prenatal care in the first trimester of pregnancy has remained about the same since 1979. Seventy-five percent of pregnant women began prenatal care in the first trimester of pregnancy, declining slightly from 76% in 1988. The proportion of mothers who receive third trimester or no care has remained at about 6% since 1983. Differences between white and black mothers beginning prenatal care in the first trimester are striking. While 79% of white mothers begin prenatal care in the first trimester, only 60% of black mothers do so. Black mothers were also 2.4 times more likely to receive late or no care than white mothers. The data also reveal a strong association between the education of the mother and the time that she begins prenatal care. The lower the education, the greater the risk of inadequate prenatal care.

LOW BIRTH WEIGHT

The rate of low birth weight babies increased slightly between 1988 and 1989 from 6.9 to 7.0%, the highest level observed since 1978 when the rate was 7.1.

The differential between the incidence of black and white low birth weight babies remains substantial. In 1989, 5.7% of white babies were born weighing 2500 grams or less, while 13.2% of black babies were low birth weight. The rate for black babies has actually *increased* steadily over the last 5 years, from 12.4% in 1984 to its present high. More low birth weight babies are surviving due to new technological developments and refinement of currently used treatment modalities. However, there has been very little success in prevention.

MATERNAL DEATHS

In 1989 a total of 320 women died of maternal causes; a rate of 7.9 per 100,000 births, a decrease from 8.4 in 1988 (2). Black women have a higher risk of dying in childbirth than white women. In 1989 the mortality rate for black women was 18.4 per 100,000 births, or 3.3 times the rate of 5.6 for white women.

INFANT DEATHS

In 1989 there were 39,655 infant deaths under one year of age, a rate of 9.8 per 1000 live births, down from 10.0 in 1988. This is the lowest final rate ever recorded in the United States. However, the United States is ranked twenty-first in infant mortality, far behind many other industrialized nations. However, the infant mortality rate for black infants was 18.6, compared with only 8.1 for white infants. Because the rate for black infants has declined more slowly than that for whites, the difference in mortality rates has been widening. The ratio of black to white infant deaths in 1989 was 2.2:1, compared to only 1.8:1 in the early 1970s.

Infant mortality can be further divided into neonatal mortality, or deaths during the first 28 days after birth, and postneonatal mortality. In the United States and other industrialized countries, neonatal mortality is largely a consequence of prenatal and intrapartum problems, while postneonatal mortality is largely attributable to social and environmental causes occurring after birth. The neonatal mortality rate in 1989 was 6.2 per 1000 overall. For white infants neonatal mortality was 5.1 and for black infants it was 11.9. The post-neonatal mortality rate was 3.6, with 2.9 for white babies and 6.7 for black babies, nearly 2.5 times that of whites. The greater disparity in postneonatal mortality reflects the greater economic disadvantages of blacks compared to whites.

More than one half (54%) of all infant deaths were caused by the following: congenital anomalies, sudden infant death syndrome, disorders relating to short gestation and unspecified low birth weight, and respiratory distress syndrome. Leading causes of deaths (in order of occurrence) for white infants were congenital anomalies, sudden infant death syndrome, respiratory distress syndrome and disorders relating to short gestation and low birth weight. In contrast, the leading causes of death for black infants were disorders relating to short gestation and unspecified low birth weight, followed by sudden infant death syndrome, congenital anomalies, and respiratory distress syndrome. The greater importance of prematurity and low birth weight as causes of infant mortality for black infants of course reflects the higher incidence of prematurity and low birth weight for black infants.

The relatively high infant mortality in the United States and the continued racial disparity in infant deaths and low birth weight is a cause of great concern for everyone. It is linked to a variety of factors including the following: the effects of poverty on childbearing women and their infants, access to and the use of quality prenatal care and the health care system as a whole, nutrition, education achieved, and the use of alcohol and illicit drugs during pregnancy. Infant mortality and low birth weight are approached as a "medical problem." There is a strong movement to provide high technology care for infants born with health problems. In recent years there has been growing attention to increasing access to prenatal care or other preventive health care programs and projects. At the same time there is very little attention paid to changing those underlying factors that would bring about changes in infant mortality such as economic stability, education, job training, decent and safe housing, and the toxic effects of toxic substances in the work and living environment.

PLACE OF BIRTH AND NURSE MIDWIVES

Hospital deliveries by physicians continue to be the predominant mode of birth in the United States. In 1989, 98.8% of all babies were born in hospitals, 0.35% in freestanding birth centers, and 0.68% at home. About 96% of births were attended at delivery by a physician, and only 3.7% were attended by midwives. Of the births by midwives, 13.9% of the deliveries were done in either a freestanding birth center or a residence, 85% in hospitals, and the remaining few in a clinic, doctor's office, or unspecified place.

As of 1989 statistics are being kept on the specific place of birth such as freestanding birth centers, residence or other non-hospital site. The newly revised birth certificate also provides more detail on the person attending the birth. Doctors of Medicine (M.D.s) and Doctors of Osteopathy (O.D.s) are identified separately. Midwives are identified as certified nurse-midwives or "other" midwives, which includes lay midwives and nurse-midwives not certified. This new information gives a clearer picture of midwifery practice. However, the number of midwife deliveries may be greater than reported because birth certificates may be signed by physicians or another designated person even though the birth was attended by a nurse-midwife.

Although deliveries by physicians continue to predominate, there has been a three-fold increase in the number of midwife-attended deliveries since 1980. This small but growing percent reflects the increased number of midwives in the United States, approximately 4000 at present, as well as their greater acceptance by consumers and professionals as competent care givers for mothers and infants. Demand for nurse-midwives exceeds the supply as more and more physicians opt out of obstetrical services because of liability issues and related escalating insurance rates. Because of this great demand, salaries for nurse-midwives have increased dramatically over the past few years. To meet this undersupply, the American College of Nurse Midwives has initiated a campaign which has set a goal to have 10,000 nurse-midwives by the year 2000.

HEALTHY PEOPLE 2000 and MATERNAL/CHILD HEALTH

The United States does not have a national health plan. However, it has developed a national strategy for improving the health of the country over the next 10 years called "Healthy People 2000: National Health Promotion and Disease Prevention Objectives." The goals of this strategy are to increase the span of healthy life, to reduce health disparities and to achieve access to preventive services for all Americans (5).These objectives include (a) significant reductions in preventable disability and death, (b) enhanced quality of life, and (c) reduction of the disparities in the health status of vulnerable populations within the country. They follow and build on a document called "Promoting Health/ Preventing Disease: Objectives for the Nation for 1990," which grew out of a health strategy initiated in 1979 with the publication of "Healthy People: The Surgeon General's Report on Health Promotion and Disease Prevention" (6).

Over one half (170) of the 300 Objectives in Healthy People 2000 relate in some way to mothers and children. Those that are most directly relevant include nutrition, oral health, immunization and infectious diseases, physical activity and fitness, family planning, reduction of violent and abusive behavior, educational and community based programs, and specific disease entities such as chronic disabling conditions.

One section specific to Maternal Child Health contains Health Status and Risk Reduction Objectives that target reductions in infant mortality low birth weight babies, severe complications of pregnancy, cesarean sections, and the use of alcohol, tobacco, and illegal drugs. Services and prevention objectives in this same section address preconception counseling, increased prenatal care in the first trimester, increase in breastfeeding, genetic counseling, risk appropriate care, and primary care services for babies up to 18 months of age (7).

FUNDING FOR MATERNAL/ CHILD HEALTH SERVICES

Health insurance or the lack of it will determine where a pregnant woman will receive care. Those with private health insurance, which is usually job-related (herself or her spouse), receive care from private physicians or nurse - midwives. Reimbursement for their services may be through a number of private insurance programs, including Health Maintenance Organizations.

For those women and infants who are uninsured, maternal and child health services are funded through multiple programs. The two most important are the Title V Maternal/Child Health Block Grant and Title XIX, sometimes called Medical Assistance or Medicaid. Funded primarily through a federal/state match, local governments also supplement these major programs with general tax funds. Administration is based in state or local government structure, and reimbursement for services takes place through agency contracts or provider agreements. This state administration and partial state funding has led to substantial variation in the way the programs are administered, including who is entitled to receive services, who can provide services, and how reimbursements are handled. Maternity services funded by these programs may be provided through hospital clinics, community health centers, or, in some cases, obstetricians or nurse-midwives and pediatricians in private practice who are willing to take part in publicly funded programs.

Reimbursement for services given may go directly to the administrative unit of the hospital, health center, or corporation that administers the program, who then pays the providers of care a salary. In other cases payment goes directly to the obstetrician, nurse-midwife, pediatrician, or nurse practitioner delivering the services. There are also some Medicaid HMO Case Management models paid on a capitation (per month basis).

Many features of publicly funded maternal-child health programs have discouraged private providers from participation. Reimbursement systems are often cumbersome, requiring multiple forms and delayed reimbursement time, causing a great deal of frustration and discontent. Except for some community health centers that are reimbursed at cost, publicly funded programs reimburse with a set fee that is often below the cost of providing care. For this reason, many private physicians choose not to care for pregnant women and infants in publicly funded programs. In addition, obstetricians must pay large sums of money for malpractice insurance. They feel that poor women, because of their high risk status, are more likely to have a poor outcome in pregnancy and sue the physician. Even though studies have discounted this, the fear remains (8).

TITLE V

Title V, the only federal program devoted exclusively to maternal and child health, was originally enacted into law in 1935 with the objective of improving the health of all mothers and children. It is a federal-state partnership implemented at the state level, currently requiring states to match $3 for every $4 allocated by the federal government. A 1981 amendment to Title V consolidated several categorical health programs for women and children into one Block Grant from the federal government. This meant that instead of the federal government's funding programs by categories, the states would receive one "block" of money which they could allocate according to identified needs. The MCH Block Grant was again radically amended in 1989. Some of the mandates are as follows: a statewide needs assessment that would identify the need for preventive and primary care services for pregnant women and infants up to age one; preventive and primary care services for children; family-centered, community based, coordinated care services for children with special health care needs; and an overall state plan for meeting identified needs. All of the state plan goals and objectives have to be linked with Healthy People 2000 National Health Objectives. The new amendments are more directive in program expectations and accountability (9, 10).

The second major program that funds MCH is called Medicaid which is also a federal/state program that reimburses providers of care for medical services for low income persons who meet eligibility criteria. These criteria are set by each state according to broad federal guidelines. States also determine the amount, duration, and scope of services. However, since 1984 there have been several amendments to Medicaid that have broadened eligibility criteria and expanded services for pregnant women and children. States are now mandated to cover certain low income pregnant women and children up to age 6 with family incomes up to 133% of the poverty level. The 1990 amendments mandate a phase-in by the year 2000 of children up to the age of 19 who are below the federal poverty level.

An important milestone for nurses in the 1989 Medicaid amendments is that state Medicaid plans must cover services of certified pediatric nurse practitioners or family nurse practitioners practicing within the scope of state law, regardless of whether they are under the supervision of or associated with a physician.

One of the Federal mandates for both Title V and Title XIX is coordination and the development of cooperative arrangements between the two programs and other state health agencies. Some problematic areas are eligibility based on income, services which the state elects to cover with either program, provider reimbursement, reporting, and availability of MCH services (11).

OTHER FEDERAL MATERNAL AND CHILD HEALTH PROGRAMS

Other Federal programs that provide services and funding for medically undeserved populations are special grants to community and migrant health centers. These latter serve seasonal workers as they follow the harvest. Because they are migratory, women and children in this population have very little continuity of care. Many do not have adequate prenatal or birth care (12).

The Women Infants and Children (WIC) program was designed to "Make available supplemental foods to pregnant and lactating women and to infants who are determined by competent professional authority to be at nutritional risk because of inadequate nutrition and inadequate income" (13). Nutritious supplemental food and nutrition education are provided at no cost to low-income pregnant, postpartum, and breastfeeding women and to infants up to their fifth birthday. Administered through the Department of Agriculture, it is implemented at the state level (14).

SUMMARY

Even though there is growing awareness of the United States' high infant mortality, low birth weight babies, and the plight of poor and low income women in our country, many serious barriers of access to maternal-child health care remain. These may be financial, cultural, or attitudinal. Specific barriers include a lack of care providers willing to serve low income or rural populations, lack of day care services for other children, transportation, and numerous factors related to poverty and the lack of health insurance. Partial solutions come piecemeal through amendments to Title V, Title XIX, and other federal-state programs. However, there will be no final solution until our federal government legally mandates that there will be universal access to health care for all mothers and children.

REFERENCES

1. *Advance report of final natality statistics, 1989,*. The National Center for Health Statistics Vol. 40, No. 8, Supplement, December 12,1991.
2. *Advance report of final mortality statistics, 1989*. The National Center for Health Statistics Vol. 40, No. 8, Supplement 2, January 7,1992.
3. National Center for Health Statistics (1991). *Monthly Vital Statistics Report*, Vol. 40, No. 8, 1-55.

4. *Beyond Rhetoric: A new American agenda for children and families.* (1991). Final report of the National Commission on Children. U.S. Government Printing Office, Washington, D.C. p. 82-83.
5. Office of Disease Prevention and Health Promotion. (1990). *Healthy People 2000.* (DHHS Publication No. (PHS) 90-50212). Washington D.C.: U.S. Government Printing Office.
6. Office of the Assistant Secretary for Health and the Surgeon General. (1979). *Healthy People: The surgeon generals report on health promotion and disease prevention.* (DHEW (PHS) Publication No. 79-55071).Washington D.C: U.S. Government Printing Office.
7. Office of Disease Prevention and Health Promotion. (1990). Chapter 14. *Healthy People 2000.* (DHHS Publication No. (PHS) 90-50212). Washington D.C.: U.S. Government Printing Office.
8. Feldman, Laura S. (Ed). (1991). *Improving access to maternity provider participation in medicaid.* pp. 20-21. Washington D.C.: American College of Obstetricians and Gynecologists.
9. Subtitle C-Maternal and Child Health Block Grant Program. Sec. 6501. Section 501 and 502 of the Social Security Act (42 U.S.C. 701) amendments (1989)
10. Association of Maternal and Child Health Programs. (1991). *Making a difference: A report on Title V maternal and child health services programs' role in reducing infant mortality* . Washington D.C.: AMCHP.
11. Association of Maternal and Child Health Programs. (1990). *Medicaid: MCH related federal programs: Legal handbooks for program planners.* Washington, D.C.: AMCHP
12. Association of Maternal and Child Health programs. (1991). *Community and migrant health centers: MCH related federal programs: Legal handbooks for program planners.* Washington D.C.: AMCHP.
13. Public Law 92-433, 17(f) (2).
14. Association of Maternal and Child Health Programs (1991). *The supplemental food program for women, infants and children (WIC): MCH related federal programs: Legal handbooks for program planners.* Washington D.C.: AMCHP.

10

Women's Health Status in the United States: An Immigrant Women's Project

Collaborating Centre for Research and Clinical Training in Nursing
University of California at San Francisco
School of Nursing

Afaf I. Meleis, Patricia A. Omidian, Juliene G. Lipson

The Mid East S.I.H.A. Project[7] is a primary health care/health resource center for Middle Eastern immigrants located in the School of Nursing at the University of California, San Francisco (UCSF). This interdisciplinary project is staffed by faculty and graduate students in the International/Gross-Cultural Nursing and Medical Anthropology Programs at the UCSF and representatives of the Arab-American and Iranian communities of the San Francisco Bay Area. With an emphasis on low-income women, the Project provides health information, cultural and language interpretation, referral services, health promotion workshops, health information, and opportunities for value clarification for immigrants and their families. The Project also serves health care providers by providing cultural interpreters and by giving in-service training on cross-cultural issues and coping styles in illness.

---

[7]The senior author was partially supported by a Kellogg International Fellowship.

With the support of a Kellogg International Fellowship, the Project developed a series of health education workshops based in the Arab-American community. Called "Being Healthy, Thinking Healthy, Staying Healthy," the workshops were held in the Spring of 1988 at an Arab community center. The focus was on culturally appropriate self-care and health promotion.

The overall goal of the health maintenance/promotion program was to empower women to take responsibility for their own health and that of their families through value clarification and a greater awareness and understanding of their own roles. The program offered a forum for immigrant women to develop skills needed to cope with the difficulties and stressors of living and raising families in a new country, with an emphasis on mastering various roles and coping with new role demands. In addition to affording opportunities for dealing with existing issues related to physical and mental health, the series provided an opportunity to discuss and demonstrate preventive measures with regard to common risk factors in the community. The Arab community participated by choosing the topics, identifying resources and information available in their area, and helping to organize the workshops.

This report describes this series and is intended to provide clinicians with a model for developing and implementing a community-oriented health promotion program based on the health needs of a dispersed ethnic community. It is based on existing health education methods for reaching immigrant and migrant women (Thompson, Harminder, & Mroke, 1986; Ellis, Stoker, & Wood, 1987; Lee & Brentnall 1986) and on the principle of community participation that is promoted by the WHO/UNICEF 1978 Alma Ata Declaration. Our model conceives health educators as facilitators who help the community to choose its own focus and articulate its own needs and to plan and implement health services to meet these needs. After describing the Arab-American community and its health to provide the context we describe the theoretical framework and the process of program development. The program itself consisted of eight 90-minute sessions on the following topics: raising adolescents, handling stress, self-care, nutrition, AIDS, child safety, employment, and menopause. Attendance varied from 5 to 35 women. The series marked a turning point for health education in the Arab community in that it not only built on previous health education requests but also offered the women a chance to actively plan and participate in a primary health promotion program.

ASSUMPTIONS AND THEORETICAL FRAMEWORK

The assumptions on which the program was developed include the following:

1) Language and cultural barriers negatively impact access to health care services. Immigrant women face particular problems locating appropriate services, arranging transportation and dealing with the structure of our complex

health and social service systems. Speaking English does not necessarily mean that immigrant women can clearly communicate their needs to health professionals. Mutual understanding is impeded by differences in nonverbal communication style and the different meanings clients and providers attribute to illness. Health and illness are defined in cultural terms and illness is a social event, a social creation that is interpreted within the social network before treatment is sought (Freidson, 1970).

2) Because immigrant women are the conservators of their family's health, their role in health promotion is critical. They make decisions regarding health care use and subsequent actions for all members of the family (Meleis & Rogers, 1987), using cultural definitions to filter information received by health care providers. Immigrant women need opportunities to discuss health topics in an environment that permits clarification of values, identification of options and resources, and the range of culturally acceptable choices. Although Western biomedicine places ultimate responsibility for health on the individual, the ability to make choices about one's everyday life is constrained by one's cultural values and limits. When information is presented in a culturally appropriate manner and is accessible and acceptable to the individual, she can better use it to make choices about health and health care.

3) Community members are aware of their community's needs and can communicate these needs when and if given the opportunity to do so. This assumption is based on principles of "community-oriented primary health care" (WHO, 1978; Newell, 1975), in which active community participation provides the groundwork for self-empowerment on a number of levels: individual, family, and community. The proceedings of the WHO conference at Alma Ata stated that "Primary Health Care addresses the main health problems identified by the community, providing promotive, preventive, curative, and rehabilitative services accordingly" (WHO, 1978). Needs are identified and then addressed through mobilization of resources within the community whenever possible. This is an action-oriented process by which the community empowers itself at a local political level (Werner, 1977). Empowerment of individuals occurs within the context of the social group, whether it be family, extended family, or community.

The theoretical framework on which the health maintenance/promotion series was based includes concepts of role, transition, self-care and ethnic identity. A role is:

> a designated reciprocity in which an interaction or a social exchange occurs and is seen in terms of relevant other roles. The role that the actor elects to play is derivative of his voluntary actions that are motivated by returns expected, and, indeed, received from others (Meleis, 1975, p. 265).

Women's roles can be analyzed as an aggregation of tasks, sentiments, and goals which are organized in coherent units in response to individual, family, and social expectations, e.g. , mother, wife, friend, and health provider. Any changes in expectations, conditions surrounding roles, or symbols within roles cause stress and subsequently may influence health or health-seeking behavior. It is important to consider women's roles in terms of the balance between the stresses and the satisfactions in each. Most immigrant women perceive their role in the context of their families (Meleis & Rogers, 1987); the dominant U.S. emphasis on individualism is not valued.

Transition is a passage from one life condition or status to another and can be developmental or situational. Transition involves both the process and outcome of the passage. A pervasive characteristic is "disconnectedness," but its meaning to any individual influences the outcome (Chick & Meleis, 1988). Immigrant women experience role changes in coping with cultural differences in the new country as well as in personal and family development. Transition includes modifying or adding roles when changes occur between the individual and her social network or cultural setting. Value clarification is helpful in allowing the individual to adapt to the new role or roles through knowledge of what the role entails. Role transition involves the acquisition of new knowledge and skills, incorporating value clarification to complete the process (Chick & Meleis, 1988; Swendsen & Meleis, 1978). Self-care focuses on health promotion and disease prevention through education. Fundamental to the workshop series, the self-care model is based on the premise that

> individuals have the ability to influence their health and to participate in their health care. Self care is defined here as those activities initiated or performed by an individual, family, or community to achieve, maintain, or promote *maximum* health potential (Steiger & Lipson, 1985).

The workshop series for immigrant women emphasized family and community aspects of self-care and health promotion.

Ethnicity, another component of the model, must be considered when working with immigrant women. Immigrants do not drop their cultural baggage at the entry gate, but pass it on to their children and subsequent generations; thus, we must distinguish between immigrant status and ethnic identity. Ethnic groups are "categories of ascription and identification by the actors themselves" (Barth, 1969) and share such cultural patterns as marriage practices, food styles, and religion, as well as concepts of health and illness. Ethnic identity is a subjective sense of belonging to a group that is distinguishable from other social groups. It includes an answer to the question "who am I?" and feelings about oneself in relation to others.

THE CONTEXT: DEMOGRAPHICS, HISTORY AND HEALTH

According to the 1980 census, San Francisco's population of 678,974 is 58% white, 13% black, 22% Asian/Pacific Islanders, 0.5% Native Americans, and 7% other. Twelve percent of the white category identified themselves as Hispanic and 0.7% as Middle Eastern (about 4800 individuals). Continuing decline in the city's white and black populations and continuing growth in the Hispanic and Asian/ Pacific Island groups is predicted.

In San Francisco, ethnically designed health and social services exist for immigrants in neighborhoods where there are high concentrations of particular groups, e.g., the On Lok Senior Center in Chinatown and the Mission Community Health Center for Hispanics. Arab-Americans, in contrast, are dispersed and heterogeneous. They come from Egypt, Saudi Arabia, North and South Yemen, the United Arab Emirates, Lebanon, Jordan, Syria, Kuwait, Iraq, and Israel. No services existed to meet their specific culturally based needs until the Mid-East S.I.H.A. Project was established in 1982. Although many Arab-Americans have health insurance, services are often improperly utilized, such as using emergency rooms as primary clinics, or underutilizing private services where co-payment is required (Omidian & Rainey, 1987).

Arabs came to the United States in several waves. The first wave (late 19th Century to WWII) consisted mainly of Christian men who sought economic gain in the New World and who never intended to stay, but eventually settled and brought over wives and other family members (Elkholy, 1966, p. 83). many prominent Bay Area Arab-American families are descended from these early immigrants. Subsequent immigration waves (mid-1940s to present) were associated with changes in the political climate in the Middle East and the establishment of Israel. These immigrants included the intellectual elite and skilled professionals, as well as refugees from the wars in Lebanon. A large number of the most recent immigrants are Moslem (Reizian & Meleis, 1985).

Currently, there are an estimated 2 to 3 million Arab immigrants in the United States. Most came from Israel and the Occupied Territories, Lebanon, North Yemen, Iraq, and Egypt (Meleis & Sorrell, 1981). According to estimates from community leaders, approximately 100,000 Arab-Americans live in the San Francisco Bay Area, and of these, at least 30,000 are Palestinians. These estimates include second and third generations while the census counts only the foreign born. Palestinians, in particular, count all descendants; those from Ramallah keep records, family trees, and directories of all who live in the United States.

Although Arab-Americans maintain many traditional values in the home, in public they are not visually distinguishable from the rest of the population. Cultural patterns and ethnic symbols remain private and are manifested publicly only in times of crises, such as illness and hospitalization.

Some Arab cultural characteristics and values create potential conflict for patients in the United States health care system, such as group rather than individual orientation, the desire to keep some information private, a belief in the primacy of God's Will, and concern for maintaining the family's honor (Lipson & Meleis, 1985). While such values are maintained in various degrees by most Arab-Americans, they are unspoken; however, they affect both patients and their families.

Illness is viewed by Arab-Americans in physical, emotional, behavioral, and spiritual terms (Maloof, 1982). Physical is not separated from psychological, nor is illness defined as a problem with a specific organ system. The experiences of pain and illness tend to be global and generalized (Meleis, 1981; Lipson & Meleis, 1985). A person is considered sick when he or she is no longer able to function or fulfill her or his roles (cf., Apple, 1960; Gallagher, 1976).

Related to the concept of illness are two symbolic categories: 1) the evil eye, and 2) balance of hot and cold. The evil eye is found throughout the Middle East and Latin America. The "eye," which is believed to cause illness, is thought to result from another person's envy or attempting to control the future. Ill effects of the "eye" can be prevented by 1) not attempting to plan for the future; 2) minimizing attention to good fortune, health and children by avoiding direct recognition and compliments; and 3) by calling for God's blessing or touching wood when compliments are made (Sachs, 1983).

Maintaining balance in the body and the environment is another aspect of the Arab view of health. People maintain balance by avoiding sudden changes in temperature and eating a balanced diet according to the season. Hot and cold foods (perceived quality rather than temperature of food) are seen to cause illness when eaten inappropriately or have the ability to bring the body back into balance if properly mixed (Lipson & Meleis, 1985; Maloof, 1982; Meleis, 1981).

In the case of illness, misunderstanding between Arab clients and health providers is due to conflicting expectations: clients expect to be cared for and health providers expect from clients some degree of self-care and share of the responsibility for getting well (Meleis, 1988). Although Arabs perceive their health to be under God's control, they also see Western biomedicine as powerful and expect immediate results from treatment. Self-care models do not make sense in this context. One might observe a person with diabetes drinking cola or a person with asthma smoking; the individual may not understand the relationship between food or smoking and health or think that his fate is determined by God, no matter what he does.

The Western biomedical model assumes a future orientation and a positive attitude toward prevention while some Arab clients have a strictly present orientation. Such value conflicts appear to inhibit the acceptance of health promotion but in reality do not really do so. Self-care is valued, but within a traditional context (protection from the "evil eye" and balancing hot and cold foods). The health promotion program had to consider these beliefs in order to be effective. In short, any health promotion program in an immigrant/ethnic community must incorporate health beliefs and behavior by using the traditional system as the context for introducing new information.

PROGRAM

The goal of the program was to empower women to maintain/promote their own and their children's health. At each session women were given a list of community resources and health promotion materials pertinent to the evening's topic in English and Arabic whenever possible. The following sessions were held.

What Are the Barriers to Happiness in America; Handling Life as an Immigrant

The goal of this session was to encourage women to develop skills to deal with stress, particularly as it relates to family relationships. The session provided strategies on how to improve communication in the nuclear and extended family, and cope with family stress and ways to balance Middle Eastern and American ways. The speaker suggested ways to develop a support group when family is not available and answered questions concerning roles of immigrant woman and wife. Coping, time out, and other strategies were reviewed.

Mothering Yourself After Your Child Is Born

This session covered self-care and group-care as ways to improve or maintain participants' own health, just as they would care for family members. The speaker talked about the mother's body having special needs during and after pregnancy, why one might feel tired and depressed after the birth of the last child, and how to relieve back and other kinds of pain. The goal of this workshop was to develop an awareness of self-care methods, and we offered some basic strategies to prevent health problems, such as exercise and breast self-examination.

Child Health and Safety

The goal of this workshop was to develop an awareness of accident prevention, with a special focus on accidents and childhood developmental stages. The topics included potential hazards in the home as they relate to growing children and how to identify dangers by looking at the home from the child's level. Regarding illnesses, the speaker encouraged breastfeeding but described safe ways to bottle-feed and appropriate times to use aspirin. She also taught basic skills to meet some common emergencies such as burns, fevers, and choking.

Adolescence

Information on raising adolescents in the United States has been the most frequently requested topic from the Arab community as well as a concern of social service agencies. This workshop explored the problems teens and parents face and offered suggestions to help parents cope with adolescent children. The adolescent psychiatrist speaker described the developmental phases which occur in the teen years in the United States, what conflicts are normal, and how to keep communication open with the teen.

A goal of this workshop was to provide an opportunity for value clarification. The participants discussed strategies for dealing with their teen son or daughter; the speaker helped mothers understand the teens' conflict between American and Arab cultures and gave some concrete strategies for coping with common situations. The women also received information specific to the cultural context in which they raised their children and had the opportunity to discuss particular problems or concerns with an Arab mental health professional.

Familiar Foods and Balanced Nutrition

This workshop explored nutrition in terms of familiar categories, basing suggestions for healthy changes on the group's dietary patterns and preferences, such as eating fruit and whole grains. The participants discovered that their ethnic foods were essentially very healthy and, with small modifications and portion control, were nutritionally sound. The nutritionist speaker discussed ways of cooking favorite foods and modifying traditional cooking so that it fits special needs and diets. The women left this session with information on how to modify their families' diets in a healthy way without losing the taste and style to which they are accustomed. Those who were on special diets understood more clearly the potential variety of "legal foods" and portion control that allow them to eat familiar food and stay within their program guidelines.

Looking for a Job or Making One of Your Own

Immigrant women deal with a variety of stressors, one of the most difficult being the search for a job. Many women asked such questions as "Where do I start looking?" "What am I qualified to do?" and "How can I work and still be with my family?" The speakers covered these questions and discussed the risks and benefits of owning a business. Women gained an appreciation of the basics of job hunting in California and of the many skills they already have.

This Is Your Body: Lifetime..Wellness and Healthy Living

The speaker addressed changes the female body experiences over time, what to expect, and how to cope with some of the changes. The session covered menopause and why every woman needs to begin preparing for it before it arrives. Women gained an understanding of the processes of life changes and the physiological changes women experience, including menopause. Women were able to focus on questions concerning estrogen replacement therapy, bone-loss, and the role exercise plays in maintaining health. They also learned some basic self-care techniques, such as relaxation and breast self-examination.

AIDS: Does It Affect You?

In San Francisco, the issue of AIDS was of particular interest to the Arab community. Women wanted to know what AIDS is, how it spreads, how to keep from getting AIDS, and where could they get information. In this workshop women discussed their fears and gained an understanding of the AIDS epidemic in the United States and what it meant to them. They were reassured that AIDS is not spread through casual contact and given some strategies on how to safeguard their families.

PROGRAM DEVELOPMENT

The workshop series was developed using a four step process: (a) needs assessment, (b) planning, (c) implementation, and (d) evaluation. In describing each step we describe issues that needed to be resolved and suggest strategies that might be useful for other immigrant communities.

Needs Assessment

The purpose of a needs assessment is to understand the parameters of the community and its concerns. The process involves gathering demographic, ethnographic, and historical information on the population within its social and geographical setting. This information provides the groundwork for understanding the health needs of a community. To accomplish a needs assessment in the Arab community, two issues were apparent—deciding how to define the community and determining the appropriate methods for assessment of community needs. Ways by which communities are usually defined, such as geographical boundaries, professional interests, language, or religion, were not useful. Arabs in the United States are diverse in countries of origin, religion, and language. Therefore, we decided to focus on already established self-proclaimed social groups such as Arab women's associations.

Methods of assessment was the second issue. Demographic data is usually used to predict morbidity/mortality rates in populations for which data is available, such as Hispanics, African Americans and Southeast Asians. However, Arabs in the U.S. are not homogeneous and have not been accurately counted in the census. Neither were the usual epidemiological tools available for preliminary assessment of health care needs of a population, e.g. , mortality and morbidity data. Thus, we used a combination of sources, such as key informants, community forums, surveys (Laffrey, Meleis, Lipson, Solomon, & Omidian, 1989), and ethnographic data to obtain information on health needs in the Arab community.

Key informants included community spokespeople and health care professionals, who gave their opinions on health needs and problems in this population. Health providers' opinions included negative or stereotypical attitudes which were probably reflected back in the care of this community. The community forum approach gave community members an opportunity to express their needs directly. The identified needs formed a basis for many of the subsequent workshops. By distributing questionnaires at community lectures (survey approach) we elicited health topics that groups wanted addressed. Some of the needs brought up by community members fell outside of the health education arena, e.g., requests for English as a Second Language (ESL) classes (Lipson & Omidian, 1987; Meleis & Rogers, 1987). However, the combination of methods provided us with a general orientation to the health needs of this community.

At the first workshop, we distributed a questionnaire to get some ideas of participants' health behavior. Of the 25 women who filled out the short initial questionnaire on attitudes toward self-care, 12 answered in English and 13 in Arabic. They came from Palestine, Iraq, Jordan, Lebanon, and Syria. They ranged in age from under 20 to over 40, with the largest number (8) between 26 and 30. Seventy-five percent were married and only one had no children. With regard to breast self-examination, 25% stated they never performed it, yet 36% did it routinely. Fifty percent had never had a pap smear, but 48% had it done routinely. Eighty percent knew their weight.

Planning

The program was planned to address the health needs identified by community members and health care providers. Designed to build on local resources, the planning process utilized weekly meetings with the presidents of five Arab women's organizations, inviting their input on community needs and support in organizing the workshops. This teamwork approach was essential in both planning and implementing the series but was not without difficulty.

In addition to strategies described in the health education literature, we identified the following issues and strategies necessary for success in program planning: work to enhance trust, acknowledge the diversity of the community and avoid alignment with any one segment, and take into account connections with countries of origin. Working with organized community groups had both advantages and disadvantages that relate strongly to the trust issue. Such groups provide quick access and entry into a dispersed community once the leaders are convinced of the value of the program, and through the leaders, the trust of community members is gained. For a community oriented model of health promotion, organized groups also provide a setting that encourages community action because such women's organizations are set up by and for women.

However, working with organized women's groups can be problematic because of distrust between groups, e.g., Christian and Moslem groups. Such distrust slows information dispersal. To reach the greatest number of community members, the factions had to be recognized and incorporated. In the perceptions of Arab women, workshop sponsorship by one group would have prevented members of other groups from attending and destroy the trust of the general Arab population which had been so painstakingly built. For this reason it helped to work with as many different groups and leaders as possible, which reduced polarization caused by political factions. However, our efforts to include all club presidents resulted in slighting one of the larger groups. Consequently, their participation never exceeded two or three women per workshop.

Developing trust, although important in all working groups, is particularly significant in a diverse immigrant population. Among Arabs, trust generally does not extend beyond family and close friends, or to outside institutions. Although we were outsiders, we had gained community trust on one level. The women's club presidents had heard Dr. Meleis speak at Arab gatherings on health issues. They also knew of the S.I.H.A. Project's work in the community. However, we could maintain the trust of the wider Arab community only by recognizing and including different interest groups. In the planning process we constantly confronted religious divisions, national differences, political differences, and even subtle divisions of city/village identification among those who were born in the U.S. Thus, ongoing negotiations were necessary throughout the planning process.

Competition between club presidents required planning to minimize the effects of these differences and foster cooperation. We could never pin down such seemingly simple things as mutually convenient dates for the meeting, because there were frequent conflicts with local gatherings, religious holidays, and holidays imported from the Middle East. When one of us asked a president why dates were not worked out first, she said that no one wanted the responsibility for setting dates and then not keeping them. By leaving the choice of times to someone else, each leader would not feel obligated to attend all meetings or be embarrassed should her members fail to attend.

Maintaining trust necessitated holding the health promotion program on neutral ground to avoid political and religious biases. Community leaders and women's organizations recommended avoiding meeting in any individual woman's house, which would have caused strain on the family or jealousy. In San

Francisco, the Arab community, particularly the Palestinians, have a number of formal meeting places. Most of the women's groups used the Arab Cultural Center, and the club presidents encouraged us to use it for the workshop series, as most community members know its location. While it was not entirely neutral, this location was agreeable to the largest number of people.

For immigrants living in a circumscribed area, a good location is the local public library or community center. Churches may operate as central locations for dispersed populations, but they may not be neutral ground for holding a workshop. It is helpful to ask the women where they would prefer to meet and work toward a consensus. Non-community locations in the area may, in the end, be the most appropriate, as no community members would have a stake in them.

The final issue and strategy is acknowledging connections with the country of origin. Current events in the home country affect community members in the host country, because most have families that remain. War, strikes, political upheavals, or natural disasters, as well as religious and secular holidays, have an impact on immigrants. Just after the workshop series began, community attention focused on the strikes in the West Bank and Gaza Strip. Each week there were meetings to discuss the news or talk to people who had just returned from visits, often organized at the last minute. This competition had the greatest single impact on attendance at the health promotion workshops. Workshop participation on particular occasions was reduced because we were unable to anticipate political events in the Middle East or the religious holidays of all of the groups involved.

Implementation

In health promotion workshops, community women can actively participate in all levels of implementation. They can choose topics, and translate, type and distribute brochures and health education materials. Leaders can book space in a community hall, organize transportation, and coordinate baby-sitting and children's activities. Invitations can be sent through the organizations or by direct mail. Most importantly, the community should take an active role in evaluating the progress of the workshops. The more involved the community, the greater the impact for empowerment. In our health promotion workshops, the women were the focal point of the process and took charge of organizing the event.

In addition to the nuts and bolts of implementing the workshops, we developed several strategies for success: presence, dialogue, coaching, and empowerment. Presence involved community leadership, S.I.H.A. staff, and the use of Arabic. Presence is the physical and social attendance of both staff and leaders known to the community at large. Presence is, we suspect, what made the difference in participation. In Arab communities in the United States, workshop topics that leaders see as important draw interest and attendance; leadership support is important for garnering community attention, maintaining interest and organizing events. When a group's president did not attend a session, members of her club also stayed away. This meant that the presidents needed to make a firm commitment to the workshop series to maintain attendance. Presence also includes staff attendance at each session; both Meleis and Omidian attempted to attend each session, which demonstrated to the community that we saw the effort as valuable. When Meleis's speaking engagements took her away, fewer people attended. Some women called to inform us that her presence was important to them.

Presence is also symbolized by using the community's language. Whenever possible, we invited Arab speakers with expertise in the workshop topic, as they understand their community's values and symbols, making communication easier and giving a sense of community control. An Egyptian physician volunteered to translate health information materials into Arabic. This emphasis on and recognition of the importance of Arabic, the mother tongue, created a presence of its own. It signaled to the community that we acknowledged the importance of their roots and values. This demonstration is critical to success in an immigrant community in which the people feel misunderstood and often at odds with perceived American values.

The second strategy in implementation was dialogue. There was continuous dialogue among project staff, among project staff and community members and leaders, and among community members and leaders. Two forms of communication were used—written and verbal. Questionnaires were given out at each meeting and by this means all participants were encouraged to state what they learned and what else they would have liked included. These questionnaires became the basis for our evaluation and follow-up and a source of ideas for improving subsequent workshops. In verbal dialogue, the presidents were telephoned weekly to assess the previous meeting and plan the next. Such dialogue helped community members maintain a high level of involvement. We encouraged the organization presidents to seek input from their members and work with us to make needed changes. Concurrently we suggested strategies to maintain community interest. Some leaders waited for our calls on the Monday morning after a workshop, perceiving, correctly, that their opinions were valued and acted upon whenever possible. The dialogue between the women's groups, their presidents and the S.I.H.A. Project staff maintained the excitement and momentum of the series as the weeks progressed. Because the Arab community's attention was divided between Ramadan, Easter or Orthodox Easter, and the political events in the Gaza Strip and West Bank, without the active involvement of and dialogue with the leaders, the series could not have continued.

A third strategy for implementing a health promotion program is coaching. Coaching means orienting speakers to the fundamental goals, rules, and strategies of the event before they come to a session. For the Arab health experts, coaching included a briefing on the age, educational level, and expectations of the audience. In the audience, some spoke little English, others spoke little Arabic, but most were bilingual. This is problematic for any speaker, and thus translators had to be placed in the audience. We also discovered that several Arab-American speakers were not comfortable thinking about professional concepts in Arabic as most had been trained in the United States. Coaching helped the speakers become more comfortable articulating their ideas in Arabic.

As Arabic-speaking experts were not available for every topic, we relied on other experts, some of whom had previously worked with the S.I.H.A.Project. They also needed coaching, not just about the audience age and level of sophistication, but also on more general cultural aspects. For example, the workshop on menopause was led by a nursing faculty member from the women's health clinic at UCSF. Before speaking she wanted to understand Middle Eastern values regarding elderly women and male/female relationships as they relate to support networks for aging women. By gaining some understanding of these cultural norms, she was better prepared to answer questions on coping.

The final strategy involves the concept of empowerment. We conceived of the workshop series as a process of empowerment for immigrant women and their community. Empowerment is the process of learning and development, incorporating self-esteem and social responsibility (Rappaport, 1985). Empowerment cannot be "given;" it is the process whereby the individual internalizes the right to make decisions and accepts the self as the locus of control. We worked with the women to identify and address their health needs in order to empower them in taking responsibility for their own health and that of their families. In creating a forum where their health questions could be addressed, the workshops fostered greater awareness and understanding of (a) their own body's needs and cycles, (b) skills to maintain health, and (c) family and child-rearing issues in the U.S.

Evaluation

Two forms of evaluation are useful in community oriented health promotion programs: terminal and process evaluation. Terminal evaluations help the organizers understand the session's impact on the participants and give an overview of the process, but do not encourage the empowerment that is the basis of our model. Process evaluations are continuous throughout the program, keep it focused on the community's needs, and empower the women by encouraging them to direct the course of the program. Process evaluations provide ongoing information to the organizers at a participatory level, ensuring that the sessions are being conducted at the right information level for the audience. They also provide speakers with feedback about their own teaching and alert the staff to the level of coaching needed by speakers. Evaluations also serve to maintain a sense of continuity for the women involved, allowing issues raised to be explored further.

Process evaluations were written and verbal. As mentioned previously, the workshop series started with a short survey of attitudes toward self-care, which included questions about weight and breast self-exams. Each session was followed by a short questionnaire in Arabic and English to see what women learned, what they wanted to learn, and what they saw as important, and elicited their opinions on how to improve the series. This question, although not always answered, was a means to encourage participation and dialogue and increased the women's participation in designing programs that meet their needs.

Verbal process evaluations occurred each week when the project coordinator called various women in the different organizations to obtain their reactions and to ask what needed to change after each session. In general, the women were positive about the workshops and appreciated the efforts made to organize them. The only consistent suggestion for change was to help the women obtain better child care so that they would not have to bring children to the workshops. Even with children being watched by others downstairs, they came into the meeting room to visit their mothers and many women complained. A specific complaint concerned the presence of the man who videotaped the first session. Because we intended to use videotapes in other areas of the country, it would have been worthwhile to hire a woman to tape the sessions properly. Finally, some women thought that the topics were too sweeping to be useful and they would have liked more time to ask questions.

On the written evaluation forms, participants provided responses to the following questions:

What skill/strategy will you take home from this workshop? The women listed strategies that could enhance health or well-being or prevent illness in themselves or their family members. From the menopause session the women listed the need for awareness of vitamins and calories, exercise, proper nutrition, and positive and negative aspects of estrogen replacement therapy (ERT). Regarding self-care, they listed as important breast self-exam (BSE), exercise, relaxation, taking care of one's self, and breaking large goals into smaller ones. The stress session yielded planning and communication, self-acceptance, and resources. Regarding child safety they listed prevention, diseases, e.g., ear infection, and how to deal with small accidents. Communication was the skill noted after the adolescence session. On employment, self-esteem and knowing your own abilities were the skills noted. And finally, on nutrition, they stated "how we can eat Arab foods." We indirectly rated the usefulness and popularity of the sessions by the number of strategies noted. The three sessions that earned the most comments were menopause (7 of 12), self-care (21 of 21), and adolescence (9 of 12 responses).

What information did you need that was not covered in the workshop?
The women wanted more general sessions on self-care, stress, and AIDS. There were specific requests for information that probably reflected individual needs on which there was no consensus. They requested the following specific information:

1. Self-care: post-partum, headaches, marriage and health, more on physical and psychological health;
2. Stress: communication with husbands, marriage within immigrant communities, and communication in general;
3. Child care: information on how to handle children from 6 to teen, child abuse, divorce and premature babies, how to do CPR, strep throat, constipation, baby-sitting, e.g., who can they leave their children with, and breast-feeding;
4. Adolescence: lying, more detailed information on individual cases, and societal effect on teens;
5. Employment: finding the right job (more details), employment interview requirements, daily life of working mothers, and specific companies;
6. AIDS: how to treat it, prevention, and condoms.

How can we improve this workshop for you? On the whole, this question generated positive feedback. The women stated that the workshops were presented professionally and included useful information. They suggested more workshops, longer sessions with more opportunity for questions and answers, and improved advertisement. Some suggested involving husbands in some of the workshops, particularly the stress and adolescent sessions. One woman requested a second session on adolescents to which fathers are invited; another stated that fathers need this information more than mothers do.

Finally, speakers were asked for written feedback on the sessions. In genera,l all speakers thought that the evening's topic was significant to the audience, except for the topic of menopause, which was too narrow; the speaker suggested adding nutritional issues, exercise, and anti-smoking. All speakers thought that the handouts were appropriate and one commented positively on the consumer focus. Most speakers observed that the women were interested in the topics, were lively contributors to the discussions, and were pleasant.

CONCLUSION

The health promotion series encouraged the women to gather, as they would have done in the Middle East, without the men around. We were surprised by the strong community cohesiveness among the participants and observed relationships similar to those maintained in the Middle East, where women turn to each other for support and not, as many Americans do, to such external resources as clinics and self-help groups. In the meetings women asked questions, visited with old friends and met new ones, learned self-care techniques, and discussed a broad range of issues. Although the sessions were structured, each meeting also dramatically illustrated the importance of nonstructured dialogue. Someone always asked for more information, and many called the Project the following week to discuss issues that had been highlighted at the workshop. New skills introduced (often related to mental health and well-being) included health maintenance issues. Classes were requested on improving or acquiring skills in entrepreneurship, job seeking/interviewing skills and techniques, and when necessary, self-empowerment through English language acquisition.

Once the workshops were organized, a high level of commitment from community members was needed for all the women to travel to a central location for the sessions. While the workshops were planned for low income women with limited English skills, from a dispersed ethnic community, this initial series was attended by middle and upper income women with varied educational levels.

To date, the Project has realized its goals. In needs assessment, planning, implementation, and evaluation, the health promotion workshops encouraged community control and empowerment through dialogue, negotiation, presence, and trust. Realizing that the consequences of empowerment could be stressful, we encouraged the women to utilize traditional support systems. We also made referrals where needed for culturally sensitive counseling.

The success of this health promotion workshop series demonstrates that the principles of primary health care are effective in urban settings with a diverse and scattered ethnic community. It is only through community participation and ownership of the series that effective health education could be carried out.

REFERENCES

Apple, D. (1960). How laymen define illness. *Journal of Health and Human Behavior, 1,* 219-225.

Barth, F. (1969). *Ethnic groups and boundaries.* London: George Allen and Unwin.

Chick, N., & Meleis, A. I. (1986). Transitions: A nursing concern. In P. C. Chinn (Ed.), *Nursing research methodology: Issues and implementation* (pp. 237-257). Rockville, MD: Aspen Publications.

Elkholy, A. (1976). The Arab American family. In C. H. Mindel & R. W. Haberstein (Eds.), *Ethnic families in America.* New York: Elsevier North-Holland, Inc.

Ellis, M., Stoker, L., & Ward, T. (1987). *Health education package for women of non-English-speaking background.* N.S.W. Department of Health, Southern Metropolitan Region.

Freidson, E. (1970). The lay construction of illness. In *Profession of medicine: A study of the sociology of applied knowledge* (pp. 278-301). New York: Dodd, Mead & Co.

Gallagher, E. (1976). Lines of reconstruction and extension in the Parsonian sociology of illness, *Social Science and Medicine, 10*, 207-218.

Kieffer, C. (1984). Citizen empowerment: A developmental perspective. *Prevention in Human Services, 3*(2-3), 9-36.

Laffrey, S., Meleis, A. I., Lipson, J., Solomon, M., & Omidian, P. (1989). Assessing Arab-American health care needs. *Social Science and Medicine, 29*, 877-883.

Lee, I., & Brentnell, R. (1986). *Cultural awareness for health professionals: A training manual.* Sydney: Multicultural Centre, Sydney College of Advanced Education.

Lipson, J. G., & Meleis, A. I. (1983). Issues in health care of Middle Eastern patients. *Western Journal of Medicine, 139*, 854-861.

Lipson, J., & Omidian, P. (1987). *Afghan refugees: Community needs and care.* Paper presented at the 13th Transcultural Nursing Society Conference, Miami, Florida.

Maloof, P. (1982). *Maternal-child health beliefs and practices among Palestinian-Americans.* Paper presented at the American Anthropological Association 81st Annual Meeting, Washington, DC.

Meleis, A. I. (1975). Role insufficiency and role supplementation: A conceptual framework. *Nursing Research, 24*, 264-271.

Meleis, A. I. (1981). The Arab American in the health care system. *American Journal of Nursing, 81*, 1180-1183.

Meleis, A. I. (1988). The sick role: A symbolic interaction perspective. In M. E. Hardy & M. E. Conway (Eds.), *Role Theory: Perspectives for Health Professionals* (2nd ed.). San Mateo: Appleton and Lange.

Meleis, A. I., & Jonsen, A. (1983). Ethical crises and cultural differences. *Western Journal of Medicine, 138*, 889-893.

Meleis, A. I., & Rogers. S. (1987). Women in transition: Being versus becoming or being and becoming. *Health Care for Women International, 8*, 199-217.

Meleis, A. I., & Sorrell, L. (1981). Arab American women and their birth experiences. *American Journal of Maternal Child Nursing, 6*, 171-176.

Milio, N. (1983). Public participation in planning for personal health services. In S. C. Jain & J. E. Paul (Eds.), *Policy Issues in Personal Health Services.* Rockville, MD: Aspen Publication.

Newell, K. (1973). *Health by the people.* Geneva: World Health Organization.

Omidian, P., & Rainey, P. (1987). *All my kids are sick: Afghan and Yemeni women.* Paper presented at the annual meeting of the American Anthropological Association, Chicago, Illinois.

Rappaport, J. (1985). The power of empowerment language. *Social Poll, 16*(2), 15-21.

Reizian, A., & Meleis, A. I. (1985). Arab-Americans' perceptions of and responses to pain. *Critical Care Nurse, 6*(6), 30-37.

Sachs, L. (1983). *Evil eye or bacteria: Turkish migrant women and Swedish health care.* Stockholm: Stockholm Studies in Social Anthropology.

Steiger, N., & Lipson, J. (1985). *Self-care nursing: Theory and practice.* Bowie, MD: Brady Communications Company.

Swendsen, L., Meleis, A. I., & Jones, D. (1978). Role supplementation for new parents—A role mastery plan. *The American Journal of Maternal Child Nursing, 3,* 84-91.

Thompson, P., Harminder, S., & Mroke, M. (1986). *O.A.S.I.S. health education for immigrant women: A manual and resource guide.* Vancouver: O.A.S.I.S.

Viviano, F., & Silva, S. (1986, September). The new San Francisco. *San Francisco Focus Magazine,* pp. 64-73.

Warheit, G., Bell, R., & Schwab, J. (1979). *Needs assessment approaches.* (DHEW Publication No. (ADH). 79-472). Washington, DC: National Institute of Mental Health.

Werner, D. (1977). *Where there is no doctor: A village health care handbook,* Palo Alto: The Hesperian Foundation.

World Health Organization. (1978). *Primary Health Care: Report of the International Conference on Primary Health Care, Alma Ata, USSR.* Geneva: World Health Organization.

11

Women's Health Status in the United States: Existing Policy Affecting Women's Health

**Collaborating Centre for Administration, Health Policy
and Health Care Ethics
George Mason University
School of Nursing**

Rita M. Carty

Women's health care in the United States is affected both by the nation's overall health care policies and by recent policies that specifically focus on women. The current crisis in the U.S. health care system has a profound effect on all people. This is especially true for women, because social and economic factors limit access to health care services for women. Without health insurance most people are without health care in the United States and employer-provided health insurance impacts heavily on women because they are over-represented in jobs without benefits. They are forced to go to private insurers, qualify for Medicaid, or go without health insurance. Women disproportionately face a health care system without adequate resources to pay for the care they need.

The Public Health Service has recently launched a major initiative to redress previous neglect of women's unique health concerns. Prior to the 1980s, women's issues were not seen as a part of the overall health care agenda and were largely ignored in health care delivery and payment, medical research, treatment, education, and prevention. There are diseases and conditions which are unique to women, some that are more prevalent or more serious in women, and some that require different treatment for women. Women's unique social and economic status must be considered in discussing women's health care issues. Also at issue are women's research concerns which include minority and sex-biased research, clinical practices, and the lack of women scientists. The research agenda must address issues related to women's roles as formal and informal care givers and women's economic, social, and family status.

The current health care crisis, its impact of women, and current trends to alleviate it are briefly reviewed. Then the state of women's health policy, regulation, and legislation in the United States is summarized. The growing attention to women's health issues is an important development that should lead to future improvements in women's health care in the United States.

HEALTH CARE CRISIS

There is no minimum standard of health care in the United States. Everyone agrees health care reform is needed but no one can agree on what form it should take. Three distinct problems appear to be at the heart of the health care reform crisis (Gladwell, 1992):

1. **Health care dollars are spent unwisely.** Health care money totaled $665 billion in 1990, which amounts to $2,600 for every person in the country and 12.2% of the gross national product (GNP). The basic issue is the way health care dollars are spent, i.e., dollars flowing from employers and government agencies to medical providers and insurers often go to the wrong places, go for questionable procedures, and finish up with the wrong people.

2. **The nation's health care bill is rising too rapidly.** Since 1970, the total health care expenditures in the United States have risen 60% faster than general inflation and averaged 10.3% in the 10-year period 1980-90 (Sultz, 1991). This increase is attributed to the general inflation (5%) , an aging population (1%) , labor costs (4%), and products and procedures in the delivery of health care. Some cost controls to decrease the rising health bill include minimizing the amount of time people spend in hospitals and aggressively limiting their contact with doctors, i.e., rationing the time and resources devoted to certain types of patients.

3. **The burden of costs is shared unequally.** In the U.S. health care system, neither Medicare or Medicaid pays hospitals enough money to cover their costs. Thus, "cost-shifting" occurs, which means that the insured pay more for health care to cover hospital costs and the cost of health care for the uninsured.

Also, some hospitals under economic pressure are engaging in joint investments with providers that raise serious questions about conflicts of interest. Ventures into the construction of privately owned, high technology diagnostic facilities by providers who refer patients for those services, proliferate in competition with hospital facilities without concern for the ethical issues involved.

Access to health insurance in the United States is usually employment-based. Women and children accounted for 20 of the 33 million Americans with no health insurance in 1988 (Campaign for Women's Health, 1991). Women are more likely to work part-time and in sales, service, or clerical jobs that pay low wages and offer fewer benefits and, hence, have less employer-sponsored insurance coverage.

TRENDS AFFECTING WOMEN'S HEALTH

In response to the health care crisis, several health care trends have developed over the past decade that affect women's health issues now or in the future. These trends include the movement to make health care available to all regardless of social or economic circumstances, education and prevention to make people responsible for their own health, and the organization of groups to include women's issues in policy, regulation, and legislation concerning health care and health care reform.

Efforts to make health care more affordable for all are important because women are disproportionately affected by lack of health care coverage. In November 1991, the National Leadership Coalition for Health Care Reform, a group of large companies and labor unions, put forth a proposal to require all employers either to provide health insurance or to pay a new 7% federal payroll tax to fund public coverage. Medicaid is supposed to insure those who cannot pay for coverage, with each state making that determination. However, states are finding it difficult to pay the costs of Medicaid. Currently Medicaid covers only about 40% of the poor and states are tightening standards so that more and more women and families do not qualify for Medicaid. There is growing public support to establish a universal health care plan covering basic preventive treatment for all Americans who cannot pay for their own insurance and essentially shut down Medicaid. Medicaid will dispense $158 billion in federal and state funds in 1991 to provide health care for 27.3 million Americans (Castro, 1991). Medicare is a $110 billion program which was designed to provide decent health care for the elderly (Castro, 1991).

There are also a number of efforts to reduce health care costs through more direct controls. These efforts are positive for women as well as others to the extent that they reduce health care spending that does not contribute to better health. However, limits in health care can also harm women if they result in less access for the disenfranchised, including poor women, elderly women, women outside the health care system, and single mothers. One trend is to put Medicare on a "need" basis and limit medical procedures for very old patients. Efforts are under way to standardize medical insurance fees and forms, curb fraud, remove conflict of interests between doctors and hospitals, eliminate unnecessary medical practices, and cap malpractice awards (Castro, 1991). The American taxpayer spends an estimated $84 billion a year to subsidize medical care for mostly middle and upper class Americans. This is because companies can write off every dollar they spend on health care as a business expense (Castro, 1991). There is some political pressure to see tax reforms to eliminate this.

There is growing recognition that health care can be improved and costs contained by a shift to a prevention rather than curative system. This shift would help women, who have much to gain from health promotion, and are currently disproportionately underserved by the health care system. Prevention and education versus diagnosis and treatment means access to health care for all, with early screening, testing, consultation and preventive education to educate people to their responsibility for their own health, e.g., problems of smoking, sexually transmitted diseases, nutrition, etc. Community-based health care which is culturally sensitive and geographically accessible could accomplish much of this in a cost-effective manner and reach the people with the most need (Campaign for Women's Health, 1991)

More and more public attention is being generated to include women's issues in all aspects of health care delivery. Activist groups have organized to push women's health issues and see that women's health concerns are a part of policies, reform, research, legislation, and regulations. The Congressional Caucus for Women's Issues, Institute for Women's Policy Research, Center for Women Policy Studies, National Women's Health Network and the Alan Guttmacher Institute are a few of the groups working on women's health issues for equality, fairness, needs, and delivery. Also, many professional medical organizations have set health care agendas for the 1990s which include women's health care issues.

CHANGING HEALTH CARE REGULATIONS

The health of women is also affected by governmental regulations of health care services. Improvements in these regulations will have a positive effect on women's health. The Department of Health and Human Services (HHS) promulgates most of these regulations, covering the provision of health care and social services, manufacture and sale of drugs, cosmetics, and medical devices, and administration of health insurance, retirement, and disability programs. The 1991 regulatory program of HHS will make improvements in regulations by cost-effective implementation of recently enacted legislation and budgetary decisions, and the review and modification of existing regulations.

Women will be most affected by changes that increase equity of access to federally funded programs. Regulations will be developed to ensure uniform application of extended Medicaid eligibility for former recipients of Supplemental Security Income (SSI) and Aid to Families with Dependent Children (AFDC), which provides for continuation of Medicaid benefits after individuals and families are no longer eligible for SSI or AFDC because of increased work hours or earnings. Head Start program regulations will be developed to assure a systematic process for recruiting and selecting children to be served. Other regulations will be developed to ensure that disability programs, Medicaid services to recipients under age 21, foster care services, and education and job training programs are administered more uniformly, equitably, and cost-effectively throughout the nation. If these changes are effective, the thousands of low income women and single mothers who depend on publicly financed health care will benefit.

A second major trend in changing regulations is cost containment, which can have a negative effect on women in the short run due to limitations on health care services. "Prudent Purchase" regulations are intended to help ensure the cost-effective use of federal health care funds. The federal Medicare program and the federal/state Medicaid program represent 30% of all U.S. health care spending and greatly influence the U.S. health care system. Regulatory actions that will help ensure cost-effective use of federal funds include the determination of an appropriate, expected percentage increase in Medicare physician payments, by analyzing factors such as inflation, numbers of enrollees, changes in technology, and access to physician care. If increases in excess of this standard occur, future physician payments may be limited to ensure appropriate Medicare program expenditures. Other regulations requiring identification of appropriate treatment and treatment setting for mentally retarded or mentally impaired individuals seeking admission to nursing homes are being considered, thereby ensuring proper medical care and cost-effective use of Medicaid funds in this population.

Regulations that increase public awareness of health issues or maintain quality of health services also benefit women. HHS has undertaken a major initiative in food nutrition labeling regulations to improve food labeling information on the relationship between proper diet and good health. Since many women have the major responsibility for purchasing and preparing their family's food, these changes will have a major impact on women. Revision of regulations to help ensure greater accuracy and reliability of test results in clinical laboratories will also be important for women. Many tests specific to women's health, including Pap smears and mammogram, have been shown to have poor reliability under the current system of laboratory regulation.

PUBLIC HEALTH SERVICE AND WOMEN'S HEALTH

Perhaps the most important single policy development regarding women's health in the United States is the Public Health Service's initiative to systematically address women's health needs throughout their many programs. The Public Health Service (PHS) established a Task Force on the health status of women in

1983 and published its report in October 1987. In September 1991, the *PHS Action Plan for Women's Health* (Office on Women's Health, 1991) was published. This action plan is a commitment to and framework for improving women's health. Each PHS Agency and office developed goal conformations within the framework of the recommendations of the PHS Task Force on Women's Health Issues, and *Healthy People 2000: National Health Promotion and Disease Prevention Objectives* (U.S. Department of Health and Human Services, 1991). *Healthy People 2000* presents a national strategy for significantly improving the health of the nation in the 1990s by increasing the span of healthy life for Americans, reducing health disparities among Americans, and achieving access to preventive services for all Americans. These goals would be accomplished through health promotion, health protection, preventive services, and surveillance and data systems. The PHS Plan includes comprehensive plans for improvement in areas of education, information, policy, research, service, and treatment. Specific goals and action steps are identified to be pursued by PHS agencies and offices in an effort to meet the priority health needs of women in the United States. This Plan describes the current state of women's health policy in the United States.

The PHS Coordinating Committee on Women's Health Issues (previously a Task Force) has developed criteria over the past 8 years to determine what is a "women's issue" and define the priority health needs of women. The following criteria determine women's health care issues:

- disease or condition *unique* to women or some subgroup of women
- disease or condition *more prevalent* in women or some subgroup of women
- disease or condition *more serious* among women or some subgroup of women
- disease or condition for which the *risk factors* are different for women or some subgroup of women
- disease or condition for which the *interventions* are different for women or some subgroup of women.

PHS Action Initiatives for Women's Health include action mileposts which are defined to chart progress in meeting goals through fiscal year 1992. This is a dynamic document which will be monitored and revised as progress is made, new information is developed, new priorities are identified, and resource levels are changed. The Office on Women's Health, Office of the Assistant Secretary for Health, will monitor progress on meeting the goals and mileposts of the various agencies and offices relative to the action plan.

PHS OFFICES AND AGENCIES PRO ACTION INITIATIVES FOR WOMEN'S HEALTH

Alcohol, Drug Abuse, and Mental Health Administration (ADAMHA) will focus on identifying significant gaps in research on addictive and mental disorders in women and on developing prevention and treatment strategies that address the needs of women. ADAMHA will work to increase public awareness of the special risks women and their unborn offspring face from the use and abuse of alcohol and other drugs, especially intravenous drugs. This Administration will also work towards the establishment of multidisciplinary research teams and facilities that include female biology specialists and psychologists or psychiatrists who are experts in the fields of substance abuse and mental disorders (Office on Women's Health, 1991, 5-11).

Agency for Health Care Policy and Research (AHCPR) has a congressional mandate to conduct research related to the quality, appropriateness, and effectiveness of health care services and the improvement of access to those services. This includes studies of the effectiveness of specific medical treatment and studies of the cost, financing, and delivery of health care. Their goals are to ensure AHCPR's program of health services research addresses major issues in women's health, and that research is conducted to improve access to and quality of care provided to women with AIDS/HIV related illnesses. Current research projects include examination of the appropriateness and outcome of caesarean sections, prenatal care, decision-making in labor and delivery, hysterectomies, breast surgery, and concerns of older women, such as those with osteoarthritis, to mention a few. AHCPR also collects information on the utilization and costs of health care services which aids in the examination of women's health care issues (Office on Women's Health, 1991, 13-16).

Centers for Disease Control (CDC) will focus on reducing the prevalence of smoking among women, mainly through public education. Estimates are that 106,000 women die annually from smoking-related disease. Also, through public and professional education, screening, and follow-up, they hope to reduce avoidable mortality from breast and cervical cancer. More than 150,000 cases of breast cancer will be diagnosed this year. It is estimated that 44,000 women will die from the disease—screening could reduce this by 30%. About 13,000 cases of cervical cancer will be diagnosed and approximately 6,000 women will die from this disease—all these deaths could be eliminated with systematic screening (Office on Women's Health, 1991, 17-18).

CDC is committed to work to lower the rate of sexually transmitted infections in women, especially those that cause the costly complications of pelvic inflammatory disease (PID), ectopic pregnancy, infertility, cervical cancer, and immune deficiencies. Eight million women are infected each year by sexually transmitted infections. There are 750,000 cases of PID which are diagnosed and treated each year resulting in more than 165,000 hospitalizations for women from ages 15 to 44. PID accounts for more than 125,000 cases of tubal infertility and 50,000 ectopic pregnancies each year. Women also share an especially heavy burden of adult syphilis and resultant congenital syphilis. Primary and secondary prevention programs at state and local levels will be implemented, and screening, counseling, and clinical care will be increased. Approximately 10% of all AIDS cases involve women and 75% of women with AIDS are of childbearing age. The proportion of AIDS cases in women is rising and will lead to an increase in HIV infection among newborns (Office on Women's Health, 1991, 21). The goal is to reduce the incidence of HIV infection among women and children through prevention and intervention that targets women at risk for HIV infection.

Food and Drug Administration (FDA) will institute a workable and sustained process for establishing a women's health agenda that is responsive to women's health concerns. The FDA will participate fully in PHS-wide initiatives to facilitate greater participation in clinical research through elimination and reduction of barriers, and policy changes relating to women's health care. FDA will incorporate women's views into its policies and programs, expand collaboration with public health education programs addressing women's health problems, and build national awareness about women's health priorities (Office on Women's Health, 1991, 23-27).

Health Resources and Services Administration (HRSA) has a training goal to enhance the awareness of health professions trainees concerning the uniqueness of women's health issues. With regard to service and treatment, its goal is to ensure that the grantees funded under the Ryan White Comprehensive AIDS Resources Emergency (CARE) Act of 1990 appropriately develop and make accessible services for women with HIV/AIDS. CDC reported that cases of AIDS among women increased by 49% in the past fiscal year versus 39% for men (Office on Women's Health, 1991, 30). Another goal is to decrease the incidence of cigarette smoking among women of childbearing age through continued support of research and demonstration projects to develop and promote intervention strategies that are effective for women and disseminate knowledge about adverse effects of smoking and effective interventions. Although the number of women who smoke cigarettes has decreased steadily over the past 20 years, lung cancer now surpasses breast cancer as the chief cause of cancer deaths among women. Cigarette smoking is the chief preventable cause of death in the United States (p. 31). Another goal is to improve the health status of underserved, poor, and minority women by increasing access to primary health care and by providing quality, comprehensive, family-oriented primary health services (Office on Women's Health, 1991, 29-34).

Indian Health Services (IHS) goals include identifying issues and arriving at a consensus for an Indian Women's Health Agenda. Another goal is to raise the health status of the American Indian and Alaska Native women to the highest level possible and to deliver comprehensive high-quality health services. Also, IHS will work to establish at least one major regional Indian women's health clinic in each IHS area and focus on health services for American Indian and Alaska Native women that will result in improved health status outcomes. IHS will establish a national Indian Women's Health Activities Clearinghouse (Office on Women's Health, 1991, 35-38).

National Institutes of Health (NIH) goals include implementing fully the NIH policy requiring inclusion of women in NIH-supported clinical research. NIH has a goal to compile comprehensive information about NIH support for gender-oriented and gender-specific research, with a special emphasis on information about women's health research efforts. Also, NIH will evaluate medical, social and legal barriers to inclusion of women of childbearing potential in clinical research and to consider broader policy issues pertaining to women's health. NIH will increase research on topics important to women's health. NIH women's research initiatives proposed for 1991-92 include osteoporosis, autoimmune diseases, systemic lupus erythematosus, rheumatoid arthritis, pregnancy, fertility, maternal and child health, women as caregivers, women and aging, dementia and women, menopause, women and heart disease, women and cancer, breast cancer, ovarian cancer, women and AIDS, sexually transmitted diseases, and immunization (Office on Women's Health, 1991, 39-48).

National Aids Program Office (NAPO) will use the relationship between NAPO and PHS Regional AIDS Coordinators (RAC) to facilitate the distribution of up-to-date information on women and AIDS to the Regions and states. This will improve quantity and quality of information on HIV infection and AIDS regarding women's health. Also, it plans to enhance exchange of information between community-based organizations and public constituency groups and NAPO (Office on Women's Health, 1991, 51-52).

Office of Minority Health (OMH) will, through data collection and analysis, determine the current PHS level of activity in addressing the problems of access to health care for minority women. OMH will also work to increase access to maternal and child health programs for minority women, particularly Hispanic, Asian/Pacific Islander, and others with limited English proficiency (Office on Women's Health, 1991, 51-52).

Office of Population Affairs (OPA) will expand the focus on substance abuse prevention and treatment in Title X and Title XX programs through outreach and training and technical assistance efforts. Within the OPA, the Office of Family Planning (OFP) and the Office of Adolescent Pregnancy Programs (OAPP) administer programs funded under Titles X and XX of the PHS Act. In 1990 the OFP awarded $130 million to approximately 4,000 family planning clinics located in 10 PHS Regions. The OAPP funded grants totaling $6.6 million to 33 care programs for pregnant and parenting adolescents, and 23 abstinence-based prevention projects for school-age youth and their families. The focus of these programs for OFP is to reduce unintended pregnancy and to support reproductive health. For OAPP, its goal is to improve pregnancy outcomes and provide primary prevention education. Both offices provide comprehensive health and social support services to clients. The long-term objective of these offices is to increase the capacity of Title X and Title XX programs to reach the most at-risk group of clients, i.e., HIV-positive and drug-abusing women. Also, it intends to increase the capacity of Title X and Title XX programs to assess substance abuse and refer clients to appropriate counseling and treatment services (Office on Women's Health, 1991, 53-55).

Office of International Health (OIH) will promote the placement of women in senior, decision-making positions in U.N. organizations (WHO, UNICEF, PAHO) where they can have an impact on programs that advance and protect women's health. OIH will include women's health initiatives in new and ongoing bilateral science and technology agreements between the U.S. and other governments. OIH will also promote activities to advance the health of women throughout the world and particularly in developing countries, through the enhanced efforts of U.S. delegations to governing body meetings of WHO, PAHO, UNICEF and other appropriate agencies (Office on Women's Health, 1991, 57-59).

National Vaccine Program Office (NVP) will work to increase the proportion of primary care providers who provide appropriate information and counseling about immunization to women of reproductive age and the elderly. Also, the NVP intends to implement an immunization program to provide vaccines for women in the reproductive age group and elderly women. Additionally, it will work to develop a plan for incorporating immunization for disease prevention in substance abuse treatment and prevention programs (Office on Women's Health, 1991, 61-63).

LEGISLATION AFFECTING WOMEN'S HEALTH

The Women's Health Equity Act (WHEA) is a package of 22 separate bills designed to improve the status of women's health in areas of research, services, and prevention. The 102nd Congress began in February 1991. During the first session, two major pieces of legislation were the focal point of debate concerning women's health: H.R. 1532, the National Institutes of Health Revitalization Act, and H.R. 3839, the Labor-Health and Human Services-Education appropriations bill for Fiscal Year 92 (Congressional Caucus for Women's Issues, 1991).

NIH Revitalization Act: (1) It will permanently authorize the office of Research on Women's Health, expand its responsibilities to include determining the extent to which women are represented among senior physicians and scientists at NIH, and establish an intramural clinical program in obstetrics and gynecology at NIH. (2) The Act will codify NIH's policy regarding the inclusion of women and minorities in research and extend the policy to the Alcohol, Drug Abuse, and Mental Health Administration (ADAMHA). (3) It will establish an Office of Research on Women's Health at the ADAMHA similar to that at NIH (Gladwell,

1992). The NIH legislation would authorize an additional $50 million to be earmarked specifically for basic breast cancer and ovarian cancer research at the National Cancer Institute (Sultz, 1991). The NIH reauthorization bill requests $5 million for the development and operation of contraceptive and fertility research centers to conduct clinical and other applied research, develop protocols for training physicians, scientists and other health professionals, and develop continuing education programs for such professionals. Also, a grant and loan repayment program would be created to attract top-notch scientists to work at the centers (Executive Office of the President of the United States, 1991). It will authorize an additional $40 million for federal research on osteoporosis, including basic research into the causes of the disease and treatments to restore bone loss or prevent further bone loss. It will establish an advisory board to promote and coordinate research and education and health promotion programs, as well as an information clearinghouse to compile and disseminate information on the disease.

Labor-HHS-Education Appropriations Bill (Signed by the President on November 26, 1991): This bill increased funding to the National Cancer Institute (NCI) by $275 million and urged it to make breast, ovarian, and cervical cancer research a top priority. Appropriations to the Office of Research on Women's Health at NIH amounted to $10.3 million; another $25 million went for a new long-term study on cancer, heart disease, and osteoporosis in older women; funding was included for the establishment of a comprehensive gynecological and obstetrical research program at NIH; $2 million was included for CDC's Sexually Transmitted Disease prevention program to initiate a nationwide screening program for chlamydia in women and their partners; and $50 million went for the CDC to run a comprehensive mammography and pap smear screening program for low-income women.

Another bill, *Preventative Health Services* (S. 1944, approved by Senate on November 27, 1991) is also of some importance. This legislation would provide funding for a wide variety of health promotion and prevention services, including establishment of a new $50 million program to prevent infertility through screening and treatment of sexually transmitted diseases. The House Energy and Commerce Committee on 8 October 1991 approved legislation reauthorizing a program for grants for the prevention of sexually transmitted diseases, including $10 million for early screening and treatment program for chlamydia.

CONCLUSION

The current crisis in the health care system in the United States has a negative impact on women's health. However, there have been substantial recent changes in public policy that could have a favorable impact on women's health in the future. These changes include trends in the general society, changes in health regulations, the women's health initiative of the Public Health Service, and legislation to increase programs and funding for women's health. These changes in policy have not yet led to concrete improvements, but they are a hopeful sign that women's health needs are finally getting the long overdue public recognition they deserve.

REFERENCES

1. Campaign for Women's Health. (July 12, 1991). A challenge for the 1990's: Improving health care for American women. A report on the status of health care for women in the United States. Washington, D.C. (2175 Rayburn Office Building).
2. Office on Women's Health/Office of the Assistant Secretary for Health/U.S. Public Health Services. (1991 September 30). *PHS Action Plan for Women's Health*. Final Report. (DHHS Publication No. PHS 91-50214). Washington, DC: U.S. Government Printing Office.
3. U.S. Department of Health and Human Services, Public Health Service. (1991). *Healthy People 2000: National Promotion and Disease Prevention Objectives*. (DHHS Publication No. PHS 91-50212). Washington, DC: U.S. Government Printing Office.
4. Gladwell, M. (1992, February 6). Reforming the health care system: An American paradox. *The Washington Post*, p. A25.
5. Sultz, H. (1991, April). Health policy: If you don't know where you're going, any road will take you. *AJPH, 81(4)*, 418-420.
6. Executive Office of the President of the United States, Office of Management and Budget. (1991, April 1-1992, March 31). *Regulatory Program of the United States Government*.
7. Congressional Caucus for Women's Issues. (1991, December). *Women's Health Equity Act Update*.
8. Castro, J. (1991, November 25). Condition: Critical. *Time*, pp. 34-42.

Eastern Mediterranean

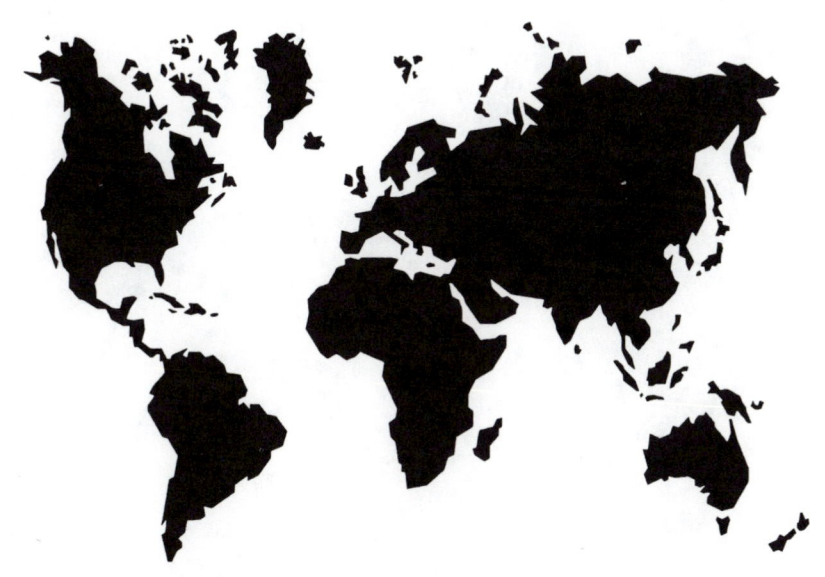

Bahrain

12

Women's Health Status in Bahrain

**Collaborating Centre for Nursing Development
Nursing Division of the College of Health Sciences
Ministry of Health - State of Bahrain**

**Naeema Al-Gasseer
Fariba A. Al-Darazi**

SYNOPSIS OF COUNTRY

This chapter presents some of the figures and indicators that illustrate the various aspects of women's health and development in the State of Bahrain. As the indicators show, women's health and development in Bahrain has grown steadily but surely. The Bahraini woman, has a major role as provider of health care to her family and neighbors.

The State of Bahrain is an archipelago of 36 islands with a total land area of 692 square km, located in the heart of the Arabian Gulf, about 22 km east of Saudi Arabia. (State of Bahrain Council of Ministers Central Statistics Organization, 1988). Bahrain is an Arab country with Muslims constituting the majority of the population. Also, Bahrain is a developing country and is going through rapid technological changes and industrialization. It faces health problems common to other developing countries, such as communicable diseases (even though there is a declining trend) and the problems that characterize the industrialized nations, such as chronic disease, pollution and mental health problems.

POPULATION

The total population of Bahrain is 488,545, with the one third of the population that is non-Bahraini comprising the bulk of the labor force. The percentage of males is 58.38% compared to 41% female. The male population is larger because of the male non-Bahrainis recruited in the labor force. The sex ratio at birth is 107.7 and the percentage of population under age 15 years is 32.9%.

The total number of marriages in 1986 were 2298 including 5.5% males with more than one wife. The average age at marriage for females is 18 years and there is a 6 year age difference between husband and wife. Some studies conducted in Bahrain suggest that age at marriage, contraceptive use, and total fertility are closely related to women's educational attainment and paid employment.

HEALTH

Bahrain's health services are free for all citizens. The life expectancy for both men and women has increased. Due to improved health services and standards of life, the female life expectancy at birth has improved. In 1988, the average number of children for Bahraini women was 5.5. compared to 6.6 in 1981. Overall indicators for health are presented in Table 12-1.

Table 12-1. Indicators Of Health In Bahrain

Indicators	1989	1981
Total population	488,545	350,798
Overall life expectancy	69.8 years	-
Life expectancy for females	72 years	67.8 years
Life expectancy for males	67.6 years	63.6 years
Crude birth rate	27.0/1000	30.5/1000
Crude death rate	3.2/1000	3.5/1000
Maternal mortality rate	0.2/1000	-
Infant mortality rate	20.2/1000	40/1000
Premature birth	45.3/1000	61.6/1000
Birth intervals (<2 years)	49.1%	-
Fertility rate	2.7	3.2
Fertility rate (<3 years)	57%	-

The per capita health expenditure for 1988 was BD.92 (US $.244). In 1989, a total of 7.3% of public funds were spent on Health compared to 6.5% in 1983. The physician ratio to population is one in 779, while there are 3.1 hospital beds for every 1000 population.

There are 19 Primary Health Care (PHC) Centers serving the population of Bahrain with highly trained personnel including physicians, nurses, and other health care professionals. Major indicators for utilization of health services by women is shown in Table 12-2.

Table 12-2. Utilization of Health Services by Women

Indicator	1989	1981
Number of births at Ministry of Health hospitals	10,165	12,000
Antenatal visits	98%	43,711
Postnatal and family planning visits	51%	24%
Hospital births by trained personnel	---	95%

The family planning services are integrated with PHC services provided at the Health Centers. In the Child Health Survey carried out in 1989 by the Ministry of Health in cooperation with the Central Statistics organization, 3623 ever-married women under 50 years of age were interviewed. The results show that the percentage of current users of contraception among all currently married women is 54%. The pill comprises 24% of all current use, followed by the condom (15%), female sterilization (13%), and IUD (4%), while traditional methods account for the remaining 44%, with withdrawal accounting for 36%.

The contraceptive knowledge of the population is very high, 98% of all ever-married women know about at least one modern contraceptive method. The pill and female sterilization are by far the most widely recognized family planning methods in Bahrain, known by over 97% of ever-married women, IUD and condom by over 90%, and injection by 81%. Knowledge of vaginal methods was reported by only 39%. On the other hand, the withdrawal and rhythm methods are recognized by 90% and 80%, respectively.

Many studies conducted in Bahrain have identified health enhancing activities of women. Studies that were conducted by Al Darazi (1984, 1987), Mohammed (1985), and Al Gasseer (1987, 1990) showed that Bahraini women are the major health care providers in the family. Therefore, it is believed that health education programs need to be directed to women, who in turn will improve their health and that of their families and communities. Those providing health education have focused on teaching women self-care.

Since many Bahraini women are reported to have iron deficiency anemia, another priority emphasized recently is the nutritional education awareness programs. Studies have indicated that 40% (Dalal, 1983) to 52% (Musaigar 1990) of pregnant women in Bahrain are anemic due to iron deficiency. Factors that may contribute to iron deficiency anemia is the short birth intervals of less than two years. The current health care delivery system relies upon intersectorial collaboration between institutions to achieve services for women.

Al Gasseer (1987) studied 50 Bahraini women's view of postnatal care, including why they did or did not follow through on postnatal visits. The Bahraini women expressed the view that only sick people visit the clinic. This view is incongruent with the health delivery philosophy and goals of the Bahrain Government in terms of health promotion and disease prevention services.

Since 1980, when Bahrain committed itself to health for all by 2000, it has become obvious that the health care delivery services are directed more toward the needs of the infant, rather than the health care needs of both mothers and infants. McBride and McBride (1981) have asserted that women's health is not only concerned with the reproductive health but must consider the over all experiences of women. In recognition of this, women's health programs have become part of the governmental and nongovernmental agencies agenda for health promotion in Bahrain.

EDUCATION

One of the major forces to change women's lives is education. The Bahrain Government provides free education to its citizens. Increasing numbers of girls are enrolling in schools and completing degrees. According to figures, the education gender gap is beginning to close (Table 12-3). Of the total population of students attending primary and secondary schools, 49.3% are female. The dropout rate for females, 1.65%, is mainly at the high school level.

Table 12-3. Indicators for Education

Indicator	Rate (%)
Literacy rate for Bahraini	69
Literacy rate for non-Bahraini	80
Literacy rate for Bahraini females	59
Literacy rate for Bahraini males	79
Female university enrollment	55
Female adult education enrollment	69
Number of nurseries and kindergartens	74

Women as Teachers

Eighty percent of the teachers in girl's schools are Bahraini. Primary and secondary school education is segregated. A plan has been implemented to educate all the teachers as university graduates with diplomas in teaching. Women are recognizing that the university degree is a key to career development and mobility.

The Gender Gap in Literacy

For males (ages 10-14) the illiteracy rate is 2.7% and for females, 10.8%; for the males in the age group above 50 it is 72.9% and for females, 93.8%. Present and future generations of females have a better opportunity for education compared to their grandmothers as the access to education is improved.

ECONOMICS

There is a small percentage of Bahraini women who are involved in businesses. Some women are also involved in "micro-enterprises" or productive activities, often in the informal sector of the economy. The women's participation in the formal economy with paid labor force is approximately 22% (21.4%). The rapid socioeconomic changes in Bahrain are bringing women into the paid labor force.

Working women are also expected to have full responsibility for children and household chores. The women are entitled to 40 days postnatal leave and breast feeding hours up to 4 months after delivery. There is no difference for retirement schemes except age at retirement for women is 55 years compared to 65 years for men.

CURRENT ACTIVITIES FOR WOMEN AND DEVELOPMENT

1. There is a process for having more representation of women at the level of planning for the health services. For example, the Directorate of Training and the Maternal Child Health Services at the Ministry of Health are directed by women managers. There are steps to acknowledge and support women's efforts in health and development.

2. The Ministry of Labor and Social Affairs offers several programs focused on the development of women, such as the productive units in which women are involved in learning crafts such as sewing. The social development projects are implemented through the network of six social centers which are

located through out the major regions of Bahrain. The social centers provide community service such as nurseries. Since 1980, the Ministry of Labor and Social Affairs has initiated a 'Community Leader's Development' program. Women with capabilities for mobilizing community resources are identified and trained to participate in programs directed at enhancing the role and status of women socially and economically. There are various vocational training programs such as sewing workshops for training young girls and women in tailoring work. The social centers are also used as places for disseminating information on health, providing counseling on social matters, and increasing women's awareness about their rights. Recently five Bahraini women have been appointed as directors at various directorates of the Ministry of Labor and Social Affairs.

3. Five out of 27 non-Governmental Agencies are Women's Associations which are very active in reaching out to Bahraini women and responding to their needs. Their main goal is to foster the development of women—socially, economically, and politically. These associations are working closely with the Ministry of Health in Bahrain, especially in the area of Health Education Programs.

4. Efforts are underway to establish a data base on women and children that emphasizes research by intersectorial collaboration between government and non-governmental agencies.

FUTURE DIRECTIONS FOR WOMEN

The key issues in women's health are to promote the role of women as change agents, make women's health and social needs a top priority, and provide women with equal access to information, technical and economic resources. The challenges Bahrain faces in women's health are the following:

1. Mental Health Services and counselling for women providers of health care both in the formal and informal sector,
2. Greater emphasis on women's health in general, especially the post natal and family planning services, and
3. The development of strategies for utilization of health services in four areas:
   - Promote the skills of health personnel providing women's health services.
   - Continue with individual and group health education for women, concentrating on the importance of regular check ups and family planning.
   - Organize home visits by Nursing and Midwifery personnel and encourage the women to utilize the health services according to their needs.
   - Promote the use of media for health education programs.

There are several strategies which can be used to develop women as leaders in health and policy decisions:
- Ensure equal opportunities.
- Train women in leadership and management.
- Provide nurseries and support services for employed women.
- Encourage membership and support services for women in leadership positionS.

The means for promoting further intersectorial collaboration include the following:
- Continuing to integrate the health education and health promotion activities with the functional literacy classes offered to women.
- Involving health personnel with various intersectorial personnel to enhance women's health and initiate activities designed to support women in development.

REFERENCES

1. Musaiger, A.0. (1990): *Nutritional status of mother and children in the Arabian Gulf Countries.*
2. Al Darazi, F.A. (1984). *Health and Illness cognition among Bahraini women.* Master's thesis, University of Illinois at Chicago, Chicago.
3. Al-Darazi, F.A. (1986). *Assessment of Bahraini women's health and illness cognition and practices.* Ph.D. Dissertation, University of Illinois at Chicago, Chicago.
4. Al Gasseer, N.H. (1987). *Reasons identified by Bahraini women for their attendance or non-attendance at six weeks postnatal visit.* Master's thesis, University of Illinois at Chicago, Chicago.
5. Al Gasseer, N.H. (1990) *Prevalence of menstrual cycle symptoms among Bahraini women.* Ph.D. Dissertation, University of Illinois at Chicago, Chicago.
6. Bahrain Health Information Center (1988), *Ministry of Health Report*, State of Bahrain.
7. Bahrain Health Information Center (1989), *Ministry of Health Report*, State of Bahrain.
8. McBride, A.B., & McBride, W.L. (1981). Theoretical Underpinnings for Women's health. *Women Health*, 6 (1/2), 37 - 55.
9. Ministry of Education Information and Documentation Center (1988 - 1989). *Statistical Summary of Education,* State of Bahrain.
10. Ministry of Health (1989). *Gulf Child Health Survey*, Ministry of Health, Bahrain.

11. Mohammed, A.A. (1985). *Traditional health practices of the postpartum Bahraini women*. Master's thesis, University of Illinois at Chicago, Chicago.

12. Planning and Social Research Section, Ministry of Labor and Social Affairs (1989). *Annual Report of the Directorate of Social Affairs of the Year 1989*, State of Bahrain.

13. Planning and Social Research Section, Ministry of Labor and Social Affairs (July, 1989). *Derasha Meydaniya wa al-sulook al-enjabifi alsora Al-Bahrainiya wa teether wasel aletesal lJamahery wa alshakhsey fitelk al mustawayat*. [Field study on levels of knowledge, attitude, and practice of family planning among Bahraini families and the effect of public and personal communication on those levels.] State of Bahrain.

14. State of Bahrain Cabinet Affairs Directorate of Statistics (1982). *Bahrain census of Population and Housing - 1981*. Bahrain Arabian Printing and Publishing House.

15. State of Bahrain Central Statistics Organization Directorate of Statistics (1980). *Statistical Abstract 1990*. Bahrain Arabian Printing and Publishing House.

16. Al Dalal, (1983). *Demographic and health variables related to pregnant mothers attending the Health Centers*, Nutritional Unit, Ministry of Health, State of Bahrain.

Europe

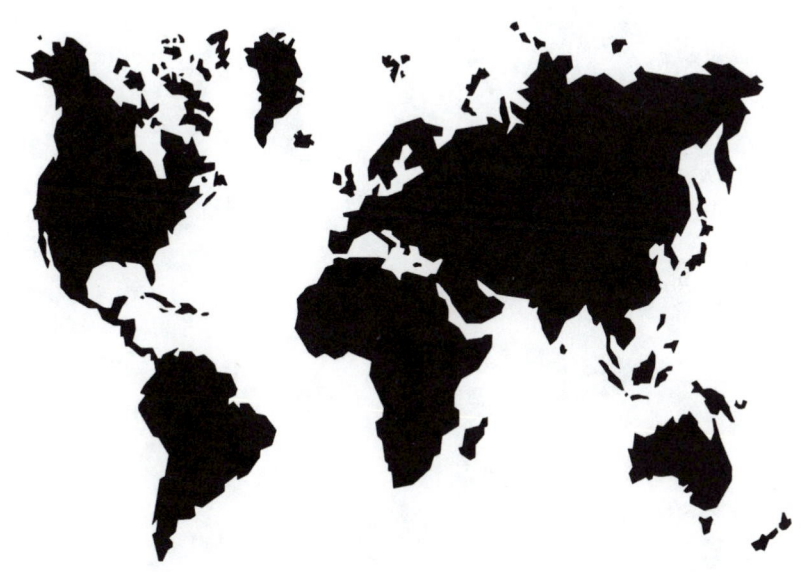

Slovenia

13

Women's Health Status in Slovenia

WHO Collaborating Centre for Primary Health Care Nursing
Maribor, Slovenia

Dunja Obersnel, Mateja Kozuh, Metoda Dodic,
Polonca Truden, Majda Slajmer-Japelj

INTRODUCTION

The basic concerns for women's health in Slovenia are 1) women's socio-economic status and equity, and 2) the complex health protection system. In Slovenia, women's health is one element of a primary health care system which includes family planning, gynecology, and obstetrics. The "dispensary" method of work has been in use for over 70 years.

Women's health in Slovenia is assessed by the following indicators: 1) maternal mortality, 2) feminine mortality and expected age, 3) feminine morbidity, 4) sick leave–absence from work, and 5) availability of health services for women. According to maternal mortality, we are among the middle developed European countries, better than the East European countries, but worse than the Scandinavian countries. Maternal death is decreasing very slowly. In the period 1970-79, we had an average of 16.4 maternal deaths in 100,000 babies born alive. In the period 1980-89, the average was 14.4. During the last three years, one mother has died each year (3.9 to 4.2 in 100,000 live babies).

Different from other European countries, because of abortion, the mortality is lowering very quickly. In 1970, 11 women died (3.7 in 100,000 live born babies) because of illegal abortion; in the 1980s, only 2 (0.9 in 100,000 live born babies). Maternal death grew because of extrauterine pregnancy; approximately 13% in the 1970s, and 23% in the 1980s (Table 13-1).

Table 13-1. Maternal Death by Cause, 1970-79 and 1980-1989

Cause	1970-1979	1980-1989
Indirect causes	14.6	28.4
Direct causes	25.6	23.6
Complication in puerperium	1.8	7.6
Bleeding	12.8	2.8
Toxaemia	8.5	10.4
Extrauterine pregnancies	12.8	23.6
Abortion	23.2	5.5

Source: Medical Report on death and causes of Death in Slovenia 1979-1989.

The female life expectancy is 76.7 years. Men live less than an average 67.6 years. Women live longer because the maternal mortality is lower and men are dying more frequently because of malignomas and cardiac diseases. Other causes of death are related to unhealthy lifestyles (smoking, nutrition, alcohol, physical inactivity, and bad coping with stress situations).

In women between 20-64 years of age, malignomas and cardiovascular diseases are the leading causes of death. In 1988, 25% of men who died from these diseases were younger than 65 years and only 9% were women. The leading cause of death among women is breast cancer (Table 13-2). Women between 19-35 years of age most frequently get cancer of the cervix uteri (24%) and breast cancer (23%); and the cases for women between 40-64 years of age include breast cancer (28%), uteri cancer (9%), and cervix uteri cancer (8%) (Table 13-3). The chances for survival have not improved; only 53% live 5 years or longer.

Observing the trends in the developed world, we can expect that in the future women will also die because of the same diagnosis as men. With effective preventive measures, it would be possible to change these trends.

The comparison between men and women in morbidity with the help of the analysis of the hospitalization is significant. In the year 1989, 143 of 1000 women older than 20 years and 131 men among 100 older than 20 years, were hospitalized. Most hospitalizations for women were due to gynecologic diseases and complications during pregnancy.

Table 13-2. Leading Primary Cancer Sites for Females, 1986

Site of Cancer	Percent
Breast	22
Skin	9
Stomach	9
Corpus uteri	7
Rectum	6
Cervix uteri	6
Ovary	5
Colon	5
Site unknown	4
Lung	4
Other sites	25

Table 2. Five Leading Primary Cancer Sites for Females, by Age, 1983-1985

Age	N	Sites	%
0-14	54	Leucemia	29
		Brains	13
		Lymphomas	13
		Bones and tissues	9
		Kidneys	7
15-39	488	Cervix uteri	24
		Breast	23
		Melanoma	6
		Leucemia	5
		Lymphomas	5
40-64	3207	Breast	28
		Corpus uteri	9
		Cervix uteri	8
		Ovarian	7
		Skin	6
65+	3822	Breast	13
		Skin	13
		Stomach	11
		Rectum	7
		Colon	7

An analysis of the eight most frequent groups of diseases (accidents, malignomas, psychiatric and neurologic diseases, diseases of respiratory system, gastrointestinal system, and osteomuscular system), reveals that fewer women (86 of 1000) then men (102 of 1000) were hospitalized. Most hospitalizations among adult women are due to benign or malignant neoplasms (18 of 1000); in adult men accidents are the major cause of hospitalizations (21 of 1000). Cardiovascular and gastrointestinal system diseases required the same numbers of hospitalization in men and women. Up to the age of 19 years, women and men are mostly hospitalized because of accidents. The main diseases in young women (up to 40 years of age) are cholelithiasis, ischialgia, and spine problems, in addition to gynecologic and obstetric problems.

Women are using more medication than men: 7.3 receipt for one woman and 5.2 receipt for one man. The biggest consumption of medications starts after the age of 15 and that is true for all groups of medications. An especially big difference (from 30% to 160%) is medications for uropoietic system, endocrinology, psychopharmaca for contagious and parasitic diseases.

The sick leave numbers in 1990 were the highest in 10 years (5.6%). This growth is greater in the female population. In 1990, the days of absence due to illness were higher in women (51.5) than in men (48.5). Men used ambulances less, but their health status was worse. The average absence was 16 days for men and 13 days for women. Absence because of the complications in pregnancy was found in 13,000 cases; the average absence lasted 292 days. Absence from work to allow care of a near relative accounted for 7%; 85% of these days were used by women and 15% by men.

Women who were absent from work usually worked in the electronic industry, in the textile industry, and in the shops. In the first two industries, the work is monotonous, repetitive, demands quick working operations. These industries could benefit from the ergonomic sciences, preventive physiotherapy, and specific health education to improve the health of their workers. Early retirement is mostly caused by diseases of the osteomuscular system. In 1990, 21.4% of accidents reported involved women and 78.6% involved men.

We are measuring the availability of the primary health care system by the number of visits to consultant stations for family planning, prenatal care, and gynecology exams, with the numbers of employed health personnel and with quality assurance indicators. During the last 10 years, every second woman of fertile age and every third woman over 15 years of age visited a gynecologic outpatient department. The curative visits have grown to 12% in 7 years and the preventive visits have decreased to 10%.

Because of the catastrophal socioeconomic situation, the number of the visits to the department is showing a slight decline, especially the preventive visits. The primary health care services for women have one physician for 9,000-10,000 women; the number has increased to 16% over the last 10 years. The number of registered nurses grew at the same time, but only up 14.5% and their number is not sufficient (1:1 to physician). Most of the pregnant women are visiting the consultant stations; the early first visits are growing (up nearly 25 % since 1981). On the average, women in all cities visit the consultant station 6-8 times during their pregnancy. In 1990, only 331 women (1.4%) did not visit a consultant station.

The vast majority of pregnant women are between 20 and 35 years of age, with 5.7% younger than 20 and 6.2% older than 35. The number of older mothers is growing slightly. The number of single mothers grew 13 % in the last 4 years. Twenty percent of all mothers are single. The level of education of mothers is different in different regions, but the majority have the obligatory general education. Regarding birth control, 10.6% of all women of fertile age are using hormonal contraception, 20% use an intrauterine device, and 4.5% of couples use condoms.

As in Western countries, the use of modern contraception is limited and therefore the number of abortions is higher. In 1989, for every 100 births there were 70 legal abortions. This is the same as in Hungary, but twice as much as in Denmark or Sweden. The abortion rate is decreasing except in women ages 30-40. Married women accounted for 71.3% of all abortions. Half of these women had only the obligatory general education. Twenty-five percent of these women aborted their first pregnancy and most did not use contraceptives. Ninety-four percent of the abortions were obtained before the 10th week of pregnancy. None of these women died.

In the mid-1970s, abortions were steadily increasing due to legislation legalizing abortions; however, in the 1980s there was a steady decline in the birth rate and the number of abortions because of the accessibility of family planning consultant stations.

CONCLUSIONS

1.   Women between the ages of 20 and 64 die mostly because of gynecologic malignoma and cardiovascular diseases.

2.   Women 19 years of age and younger require health care services for accidents more than any other reason. After the age of 20, women require health services most frequently for pregnancy related complications and diseases of the osteomuscular and gastrointestinal system.

3.   High maternal mortality is a major concern, particularly among single mothers and other women who choose to abort unwanted pregnancies.

4.   The availability of specific health services is insufficient in prenatal and postnatal care (family planning).

CHALLENGES FOR THE FUTURE

1. Health education for a healthier life style.
2. Solving ecologic problems.
3. Better development of a network of primary health care institutions.
4. National programs need to be developed with a focus on women's health, particularly preventives measure that reduce health risks (breast examinations, early extrauterine pregnancy diagnosis, etc.).
5. Availability of modern contraception must improve.
6. Politicians need to be re-educated regarding goals for health care delivery, that is, that health services are not consumers of national income, but producers of healthy populations, which is at the moment the only material source for the socioeconomic reorientation in the country.

South-East Asia

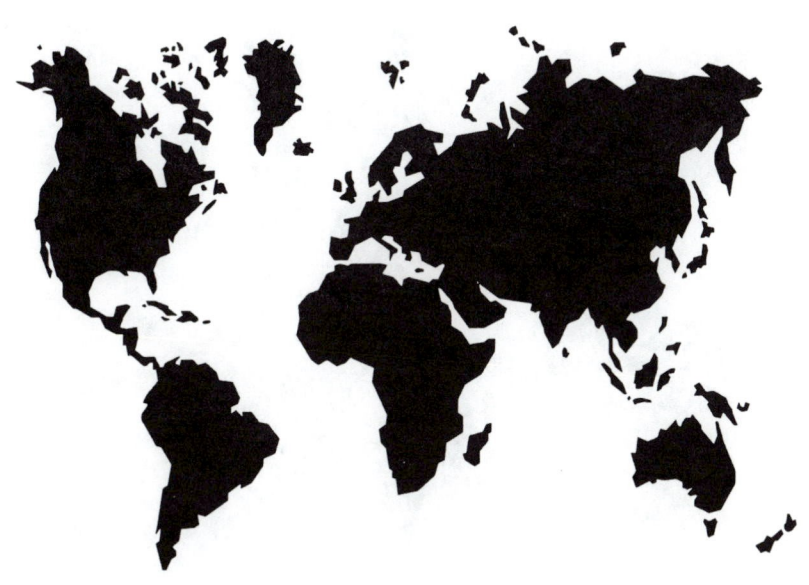

South-East Asia

14

Women's Health Status in South-East Asia

South-East Asia Regional Office
Women's Health and Development

Sally Ann Bisch

The socioeconomic conditions and health status of women in the South-East Asia Region (SEAR) of WHO vary from country to country, as do the overall conditions of countries. The 11 SEAR countries—Bangladesh, Bhutan, Democratic People's Republic of Korea (DPR Korea), India, Indonesia, Maldives, Mongolia, Myanmar, Nepal, Sri Lanka and Thailand—are spread over a vast geographical area with a tremendous diversity of land mass, population size, ecological range, political and economic systems, and sociocultural patterns. Nine of the 11 countries lie in tropical/subtropical zones. The two exceptions are DPR Korea and Mongolia, which have very different ecologic and economic systems and much higher levels of urbanization and female participation in socioeconomic and political life.

Nonetheless, several common elements predominate to characterize the Region as a whole. Chiefly, despite trends of industrialization and urbanization, it is mainly agrarian, having a traditional, sex-segregated setting that affects women's access to development inputs in critical ways. Importantly, while levels of progress and modernization vary, the countries continue to share an age-old Asian cultural ambience in which the young defer to the old and the female to the male.

Population

According to the 1990 State of the World Population Report, the global population was 5.3 billion in mid-1990. The 11 countries which comprise the WHO South-East Asia Region account for 1.3 billion people, about a quarter of the world's total population. At the global level, the sex ratio in 1990 is estimated to be 101.4 males per 100 females, thus indicating a gap of 35.6 million between the world's male and female populations. As can be seen from Table 14-1, India and Bangladesh account for 32 million of this gap. Bhutan has smaller absolute figures, but its gap spans the highest proportion of excess males, at 7.2%. Nepal, at a lower 5.4%, is nearer the Region's overall average. However, in the remaining six SEAR countries, three (Mongolia, Sri Lanka, and Thailand) have only marginal differences, and in three (DPR Korea, Indonesia, and Myanmar) there is a reverse situation with more females than males.

Structural changes in the age composition of the population are indications of a decline in fertility and an increase in life expectancy. The age group from 0 to 14 years declined from 41.5% in 1980 to 38% in 1985 and is projected to be 35% by the year 2000. In 2025, it is expected to reach 22% (the 1985 proportion in developed countries). The proportion of those in the reproductive age group is projected to go from 43.9% in 1980 to 48.7% in 2000. The percentage of the elderly (65+ years), meanwhile, is steadily increasing.

Table 14-1. South-East Asia Region Population Profile, 1990

Country	Population (000's)		Sex Ratio (Males/100 Females)
	Total	Female	
Bangladesh	115,593	56,033	106.3
Bhutan	1,516	732	107.2
DPR Korea	22,937	11,539	98.8
India	853,373	412,328	107.0
Indonesia	180,514	90,517	99.4
Maldives	200		108.6[a]
Mongolia	2,227	1,110	100.6
Myanmar	41,675	20,942	99.0
Nepal	19,143	9,318	105.4
Sri Lanka	17,209	8,575	100.7
Thailand	55,702	27,751	100.7
Total	1,310,088	638,845	105.0

Sources: UN World Population Prospects 1988 Statistical Yearbook of Maldives, 1986
[a]1986's

The dependency ratio, i.e. children below 15 years and elderly above 65 years in proportion to the working age population between 15 and 64 years, is a rough indicator of the economic burden borne by a society. Though declining, this ratio remains quite high in SEAR, averaging 1.5 dependents to every 2 working persons, as opposed to 1 dependent to every 2 working individuals in developed countries. As the care of children and the elderly is generally the responsibility of females in SEAR, it can be expected to influence their health status, particularly in the poor and femaleheaded households.

Nearly three-quarters of the SEAR population live in rural areas. However, the proportion of rural females as a percentage of total females is well above three-quarters in almost all reporting countries, ranging between 77% to 83% in most countries, 88% in Bangladesh and 94% in Nepal. Mongolia is the exception at 48.5%. Women's rural existence is, by and large, cloistered by the traditional way of life.

Rapid urbanization is, however, overtaking the South-East Asia Region. During the period from 1965 to 1984, the urban population of SEAR increased substantially. By the mid-eighties more than 1 in 5 persons in the Region was living in an urban setting; by 1990 this has increased to nearly 27%. The pace of urbanization has been fast and will continue to be so. By the year 2000 the urban population is projected to reach 33%—that is, 1 in 3 persons will be in an urban setting by the end of this century. By the year 2025 this will exceed 1 in 2 persons.

Literacy and Education

Although substantial progress in literacy was made in the Region during the last decade, disturbingly high levels of female illiteracy still persist in several countries (Table 14-2.) *Adult female illiteracy* in 1985 ranged from lows of 0% in DPR Korea and Mongolia, 7% in the Maldives, 12% in Thailand and 17% in Sri Lanka to highs between 71% in India and 90% in Bhutan. The absolute numbers signified by the high illiteracy levels for females are even more alarming. For example, Bangladesh and India account for over 24.1 million urban and over 138.4 million rural female illiterates of 15+ years of age.

Adult female literacy ratios, as a percentage of adult male literacy, range from less than one-third to one-half in countries of the Indian subcontinent for which figures are available. In other countries of the Region very high levels of female literacy ratios have been achieved, ranging from 78% to 95%. Maldives even reports a higher literacy rate for females than for males. However, despite notable success with female literacy in several countries, parity of educational achievement between the sexes has not been attained.

Despite considerable progress from earlier low levels, in certain countries of the Region a large proportion of girls below the age of 15 remain out of the educational system. Of those that join, drop-out rates are high. The following

Table 14-2. Adult Illiteracy in South-East Asia Region Countries, 1985

Country	Adult Illiteracy Rate (%)	
	Female	Male
Bangladesh	78	67
Bhutan	90	
DPR Korea	0	0
India	71	57
Indonesia	35	26
Maldives	7	8
Mongolia	0	0
Myanmar	27.7[a]	19.4[a]
Nepal	88	74
Sri Lanka	17	13
Thailand	12	9

Sources: World Development Report 1990, World Bank Bulletin of Regional Health
Information 1986-87, WHO/SEARO
The State of the Maldivian Woman, 1989, UNICEF
UNESCO Statistical Yearbook 1990
[a]1990.

figures for the primary school age group are illustrative of the extent of the
problem as of 1987: in Bangladesh 1 out of 2 girls, in Bhutan more than 4 out
of 5 girls, and in India 1 out of 5 girls are *not in school*. However, on the
positive side, Mongolia, Myanmar, and Sri Lanka report all girls below 15 years
of age are enrolled in school.

At the secondary school level, the critical base for better jobs in the modern
economy, the situation is far more unsatisfactory: only 1% of the girls in Bhutan,
11% in Bangladesh, and 27% in India are enrolled in school. Even in Sri Lanka,
where primary education has been universalized, enrollment at the secondary
level has still left out 1 in every 3 girls.

Primary school enrollment rates for females are uniformly lower than those
for males in every country of the Region except one where gender specific
statistics are available (Table 14-3). Indonesia, Myanmar, and Sri Lanka report
100% or more female enrollment. Myanmar and Sri Lanka report a primary
enrollment ratio of females to males of 97% and Indonesia of 96%. Within the
Indian subcontinent the ratio range is from a low of 45% in Nepal to a high of
84% in Bangladesh. At the secondary school level, two countries (Mongolia and
Sri Lanka) have actually achieved a higher enrollment of girls than boys, but the
situation within the Indian subcontinent is again in the range of less than one-third
to a little over one-half.

Table 14-3. Females Enrolled in School (1986-87) and Enrollment Ratios (1986-88) for Selected South-East Asia Region Countries

| | Percentage of Age Group Enrolled in Education[a] | | | | Enrollment Ratios: Females as Percentage of Males |
| | Primary | | Secondary | | |
Country	Total	Female	Total	Female	Primary/Secondary
Bangladesh	59	49	18	11	84/46
Bhutan	24	17	4	1	65/29
India	98	81	39	27	72/54
Indonesia	118	115	46		96/
Mongolia					103/109
Myanmar	103	100	24	23	97/
Nepal	82		26		45/31
Sri Lanka	104	102	66	69	97/110

[a]Primary (et al.) school enrollment data are estimates of *children of all ages* enrolled in primary school. The enrollment rate may exceed 100% because some pupils are younger or older than the country's standard primary school age.

Sources: State of the World's Children 1990, UNICEF.
UNESCO Statistical Yearbook.

Economic Situation

Although the per capita GNP has been rising in all SEAR countries, the vast majority of the population exist below the poverty line. In much of the Region serious economic deprivations subsist on a scale which, in terms of absolute numbers, is not to be seen in any other region of the world. This is coupled with ill-health of massive numbers—continuing communicable and parasitic diseases, undernutrition and related deficiency disorders—with the corresponding morbidity and mortality prevailing among women and children.

Between 15% and 86% of the urban population and 34% and 86% of the rural population in some SEAR countries live below the absolute poverty level (Table 14-4). The UN World Survey on the Role of Women in Development (UN WID Survey) estimates female-headed households in Asia at 15% to 20% of all households. Their prevalence has been noted in countries as diverse as poverty stricken Bangladesh and rapidly modernizing Thailand. That the actual incidence is likely to be much higher, especially in the most impoverished segments, can be gauged by the statistics for India, where 35% of households below the poverty line are estimated to be femaleheaded. Similarly, in Bangladesh, 15% of all rural households and 25% of all landless households are estimated to be female-headed,

Table 14-4. Population below Absolute Poverty Level in
Selected South-East Asia Region Countries, 1977-1987

Country	Population (%) Below Absolute Poverty Level Urban/Rural
Bangladesh	86/86
India	40/54
Indonesia	26/44
Myanmar	40/40
Nepal	55/61
Thailand	15/34

Source: State of the World's Children 1990, UNICEF.

while over 51% of the population are below the poverty line in rural areas and
56% in urban areas are females.

Altogether, of the world's billion poor, more than half are in SEAR; almost
one-half billion, including 300 million of the absolute poor, are in South Asia.
Within South Asia, India alone holds 420 million of the world's poor, nearly
40% of the world's most impoverished.

According to the World Development Report 1990, growth of the Gross
Domestic Product (GDP) was strongest in South and East Asia over the 1980s,
but in 1989 it had slowed to nearly half of the rate of the previous year. Even for
the period 1980-85, the rate of growth of per capita GDP was higher in only 5
of the 11 SEAR countries; in 6 countries it had decreased from its 1970-75 level
(Table 14-5). The beginning of the nineties decade has already witnessed the
development of external conditions likely to seriously undermine optimistic rate
of growth predictions in the Region, diminishing hopes for effectively making a
dent in the pervasive poverty.

Economically Active Women

Table 14-6 shows that in three SEAR countries (DPR Korea, Mongolia, and
Thailand) the percentage of economically active women is at a high level, with
at least 64% of all females over 15 years of age economically active. In
Myanmar the percentage of economically active women to all women is 50%. In
all SEAR countries except Bangladesh the share of women in the economically
active population is between 25.4% and 45.9%. In Bangladesh it is only 6.5%.
The majority of the recognized working women are in agriculture and constitute
from 30% to 55.8% of the agricultural workers in the countries, while in
Bangladesh the figure is around 6%.

Table 14-5: Rates of Growth of Per Capita Gross Domestic Product in South-East Asia Region Countries

Country	Average Annual Rates of Growth of Per Capita Gross Domestic Product (%)	
	1970-75	1980-85
Bangladesh	4.8	3.7
Bhutan	5.2	5.5
DPR Korea	12.0	9.9
India	2.6	5.5
Indonesia	8.5	3.8
Maldives	13.5	6.6
Mongolia	6.8	6.5
Myanmar	2.1	5.5
Nepal	2.0	3.4
Sri Lanka	3.3	5.1
Thailand	6.4	5.1

*Net material product
Source: 1989 UN World Survey on the Role of Women in Development.

Table 14-6. Economically Active Females in Selected South-East Asia Region Countries

Country	Percentage of Females 15+ Who Are Economically Active	Females as Percent of Economically Active Population	Females in Agriculture as Percent of Economically Active Population	Females as Percent of Agricultural Workers
Bangladesh	6.5	6.5	4.5	6.1
Bhutan	44.0	31.7	32.4	35.0
DPR Korea	64.2	45.9	23.9	55.8
India	30.7	25.4	21.5	30.9
Indonesia	36.7	31.1	17.1	30.0
Mongolia	71.9	45.5	16.3	40.9
Myanmar	50.1	37.2	15.7	29.6
Nepal	44.2	32.9	33.9	36.4
Sri Lanka	29.9	26.9	15.6	29.2
Thailand	70.9	45.8	34.9	49.3

Source: 1989 UN World Survey on the Role of Women in Development.

From data available from seven SEAR countries at the upper end of the women's work spectrum, the percentages of women in professional and administrative services range from lows of 8% and 11% in Nepal and Bangladesh, respectively, to a high of 47% in Thailand. In Indonesia and Sri Lanka the percentage is around 40%, with India and DPR Korea at 18% and 22%, respectively. Of those employed in clerical, sales, and service occupations, 36% are women in DPR Korea, 44% in Indonesia, and 55% in Thailand, but the percentages are lower in the other countries (Table 14-7).

Table 14-7. Percentage of Females by Occupation Groups for Selected South-East Asia Region Countries

Country	Professional Administrative	Clerical Sales Services	Production Transport Labourers
Bangladesh	11.13	22.56	16.89
DPR Korea	22.83	36.08	23.95
India	18.07	8.76	11.69
Indonesia	39.09	43.97	28.96
Nepal	7.93	10.24	8.96
Sri Lanka	41.06	12.62	14.64
Thailand	47.05	55.83	30.07

Source: 1989 UN World Survey on the Role of Women in Development.

Access to Safe Water and Sanitation

Lack of safe water and sanitation facilities plays a major role in ill-health. Considering women's almost exclusive role as household manager, which includes procurement of water and fuelwood, this has a great impact on their immediate environment and domestic workload. For the same reasons, women's contributions and participation in efforts to improve the availability of safe water and environmental sanitation, a crucial health target, can be substantial. According to the 1985 data, urban-rural differentials exist in all reporting SEAR countries (Table 14-8).

Deprivation of safe water in rural areas (1985) ranged from lows in Thailand, India, and Bangladesh (34%, 44%, and 51%, respectively) to a maximum of 88% in the Maldives. In urban areas the percentage of those without safe water was 76% in Bangladesh and 57% in Indonesia. Sri Lanka, India, and Nepal were among the better served urban populations but still reported 18% to 30% without safe water. Although efforts for the provision of safe water have greatly intensified over the decade, resulting in a 17% increase in safe water availability in rural areas, efforts have fallen short in urban areas in Asia as a whole.

Table 14-8. Percentage of Population without Safe Water and Sanitation
Facilities in Selected South-East Asia Region Countries, 1985

Country	Without Safe Water		Without Sanitation Facilities	
	Urban	Rural	Urban	Rural
Bangladesh	76	51	76	97
Bhutan	60	85	0	95
India	27	44	72	99
Indonesia	57	64	66	62
Maldives	41	88	0	98
Myanmar	64	76	51	79
Nepal	30	75	83	100
Sri Lanka	18	71	35	62
Thailand	44	34	22	54

Source: Bulletin of Regional Health Information 1986-87, WHO/SEARO.

In terms of sanitation facilities the plight is worse. The rural deprivation figures
touch 95-100% for Bangladesh, Bhutan, India, the Maldives, and Nepal, and are
lower, but still appallingly high, for Indonesia, Sri Lanka (both at 62%), and
Myanmar (79%). The urban situation for sanitation was better in the Maldives
and Bhutan, where full coverage was reported. For all other countries where
rural-urban breakdown data are available, the urban deprivation ranged from 22%
to 83%.

THE HEALTH SITUATION

Overall there have been some notable gains in the health situation of the
Region, though indicators fall short of the targets in almost all instances. Life
expectancy and mortality trends are key indicators of overall health status. Other
indicators, such as infant, under-5, and maternal mortality rates, women's nutritional status and incidence of low birthweight babies, as well as indirect indicators such as availability of safe water, sanitation facilities and maternal health
services, are particularly crucial in the context of limited sex-specific information.

Life Expectancy

The South-East Asia Region has experienced an impressive increase in life
expectancy since the mid-sixties, testifying to improvements in general conditions.
In seven SEAR countries, increases in female life expectancy during the second
half of the eighties were either of the same order or higher than male life

expectancy increases. However, in four countries of the Region life expectancy remained below the world average of 60 years.

Male-female life span differentials—consistent with global trends reflecting the female biological advantage—prevail in more than half the countries of the Region, ranging from 3 to 7 years (Table 14-9). They are higher than the average for less developed regions as whole (2.1 years) but far below the developed world's average for female advantage (7.8 years).

Table 14-9. Life Expectancy in South-East Asia Region Countries

Country	Male 1984	Male 1988	Female 1984	Female 1988	Life Expectancy of Females as Percent of Males—1987
Bangladesh	50	51	51	51	98.6
Bhutan	44	49	43	47	96.9
DPR Korea	65		72		109.8
India	56	58	55	58	100.3
Indonesia	53	59	56	62	105.1
Maldives	53.4[a]	61	49.5[a]	59.5	
Mongolia	61		65		106.7
Myanmar	57	59	60	62	105.9
Nepal	47	52	46	51	97.6
Sri Lanka	68	68	72	73	106.2
Thailand	62	63	66	68	106.4

[a]Data for 1982.

Sources: Bulletin of Regional Health Information 1986-87, WHO/SEARO.
World Development Report 1990, World Bank.
State of the World's Children 1990, UNICEF .

The life expectancy increases are an outcome of the overall decline in mortality, particularly infant mortality, across the Region. Gender differentials in mortality, where these existed earlier, have diminished in most of the Region. In certain countries (i.e. Indonesia, Mongolia, Myanmar, Sri Lanka, and Thailand) these have even turned to the advantage of females. only within the Indian subcontinent have the improvements in female mortality not been commensurate with that in males.

Family Formation Trends

Fertility levels have been declining in all SEAR countries, but more slowly in some than in others and from the extremely high levels that were prevailing in the seventies. Table 14-10 shows the total fertility rate (TFR) in selected SEAR countries for 1960, 1980, and 1988, the reduction in TFR for the periods 1960-80 and 1980-88, and the average annual rate of reduction for theie two periods.

Table 14-10. Decline in Total Fertility Rates in Selected South-East Asia Region Countries

Country	Total Fertility Rate			Reduction in Total Fertility Rate		Average Annual Rate of Reduction (%)	
	1960	1980	1988	1960-80	1980-88	1960-80	1980-88
Bangladesh	6.7	6.4	5.5	0.3	0.9	0.2	1.9
Bhutan	6.0	5.6	5.5	0.4	0.1	0.3	0.2
DPR Korea	5.7	4.3	3.6	1.4	0.7	1.4	2.2
India	5.9	4.8	4.3	1.1	0.5	1.0	1.4
Indonesia	5.5	4.4	3.2	1.1	1.2	1.1	4.0
Mongolia	5.7	5.5	5.4	0.2	0.1	0.2	0.2
Myanmar	6.0	4.8	4.0	1.2	0.8	1.1	2.3
Nepal	5.8	6.4	5.9	-0.6	0.5	-0.5	1.0
Sri Lanka	5.3	3.5	2.6	1.8	0.9	2.1	3.7
Thailand	6.4	3.9	2.5	2.5	1.4	2.5	5.6

Source: Sate of the World's Children 1990, UNICEF.

When reviewing the last two columns of Table 14-10, it may be seen that the average annual percent reduction in TFR increased dramatically in Bangladesh (over 9 times) and in Indonesia (over 3.5 times). Myanmar and Thailand more than doubled their reduction rates, while Sri Lanka, DPR Korea and India hastened the decline in rates by another 80%, 60% and 40% respectively. Nepal finally moved out of an upward spin to a small, but positive decline in TFR. Mongolia remained steady at a negligible level of reduction, while in Bhutan the already low reduction rate was further slowed.

The changes in the TFR itself for these countries during the periods 1960-80 and 1980-88 can be seen in columns 4 and 5 of Table 14-10. Even with these reductions, however, some countries in the Region still have fertility levels that are among the highest in the world.

According to the UNFPA State of the World Population Report in 1990, the TFR is 1.9 in the more developed regions and 1.6 in Western Europe. In no country of SEAR is the total fertility rate reported at less than 2 (1988). It is less than 3 in only two countries of the Region (Sri Lanka at 2.6 and Thailand at 2.5). DPR Korea, despite a number of health indicators on par with developed world levels, records a fertility rate of 3.6, while Indonesia reports 3.2. In the remaining six countries of the Region with available data, the total fertility rate ranges between 4.0 and 5.9.

Teenage brides are a common phenomenon in some countries of SEAR, with the average age at first marriage for females being 16.7 years in Bangladesh, 17.9 in Nepal and 18.7 in India. In all other SEAR countries for which data are reported in the UN WID Survey, the age at first marriage for females is 20 years or more (Table 14-11). UNFPA observes that, world-wide, women who marry at 20 or older have 1.8 fewer childen than those who marry before 20.

Table 14-11. Average Age for Femles and Males at First Marriage in Selected South-East Asia Region Countries

Country	Female	Male
Bangladesh	16.7	23.9
India	18.7	23.4
Indonesia	20.0	24.1
Myanmar	22.4	24.6
Nepal	17.9	21.5
Sri Lanka	24.4	27.9
Thailand	22.7	24.7

Source: 1989 UN World Survey on the Role of Women in Development.

Mortality

As shown in Table 14-12, five countries in SEAR now have Crude Death Rates (CDRS) of less than 10, comparable to developed country levels. In six SEAR countries CDRs of 10 or more persist, pointing to the continued prevalence of health problems that are well containable in the modern age. All high CDR countries are also seen to have high infant, under-5, and maternal mortality rates.

The under-5 mortality rate (U5MR) is, in particular, a sensitive indicator of the development process. It is considered to reflect the level of satisfaction of the most essential human needs in which women's roles are critical. The under-5 mortality toll in SEAR countries, as of 1988, is 5.75 million deaths annually.

Table 14-12. Mortality in South-East Asia Region Countries—1988

Country	Crude Death Rate	Mortality Rates			Risk of Dying by Age 5	
		Under 5	Infant	Maternal[a]	Female	Male
Bangladesh	15	188	118	600	175	160
Bhutan	17	197	127	770	186	178
DPR Korea	5	33	24	41	26	35
India	11	149	98	340	118	120
Indonesia	11	119	84	450	75	90
Maldives	9	91	68	330		
Mongolia	8	59	44	100	76	91
Myanmar	10	95	69	135	79	94
Nepal	15	197	127	830	187	173
Sri Lanka	6	43	32	60	19	27
Thailand	7	49	38	50	28	38

[a]1980-1987.

Note: Crude Death Rate is given per 1000 population; Under-5 and Infant Mortality Rates per 1000 livebirths; Maternal Morbidity Rate per 100,000 live births

Sources: State of the World's Children 1990, UNICEF.
World Development Report 1990, World Bank.
Bulletin of Regional Health Information 1986-87, WHO/SEARO.
1984 Demographic Sample Survey, Royal Government of Bhutan.

In Bangladesh, Bhutan, India, and Nepal, both the infant mortality rate (IMR) and U5MR are unconsciounably high, with the IMR being 98 and above and the U5MR 149 and above per 1000 livebirths, nearly six times the maximum level for developed regions. The levels of IMR are also considerably high in Indonesia, the Maldives and Myanmar, at well above the 50 per 1000 stipulated as one of the HFA goals, and with U5MRs above 90 per 1000. Four countries in SEAR fall within a middle category with under-5 mortality levels ranging between 33 and 59. No country in the Region has reached the developed world level of U5MR below 30. Further, aggregate country figures mask differentials found within a country, such as those between urban and rural areas and between different socioeconomic groups.

Maternal mortality rates (MMRS) reflect the risk to women of dying during pregnancy and childbirth. Table 14-12 shows that these rates vary widely between SEAR countries. During the period 1980-87 the MMR ranged from 41 per 100,000 livebirths in DPR Korea to 830 in Nepal. However, even in the SEAR country with the lowest MMR, the mortality rate is more than double the average MMR of 17.3 reported for the more developed regions as a whole.

At the top end of the range in SEAR, the MMR is almost fifty times the developed world-average. As fertility levels are also higher, the *lifetime risks* incurred by women in SEAR further increase—doubling or tripling, depending upon the country's fertility levels. In addition, within countries, maternal mortality varies among women of different age groups, socioeconomic categories, and levels of education. For example, younger and older women, particularly those under 15 and over 40, face a risk of death that may be 10 to 15 times higher than women in their twenties. The vast differentials in MMR have been described as "the single biggest inequity in global public health statistics." The inequities within the Region, as well as between subgroups within a country, are cause for equal concern. They reflect inadequate availability of or access to technologies and services that have been identified as fully affordable and implementable.

The major causes of maternal deaths have been identified as hemorrhage, infections, toxemia, septic abortion, obstructed labour, and ruptured uterus. Studies of the causes of maternal mortality conducted in several countries of the Region have shown that anemia, repeated pregnancies, and pregnancies at very young ages are important predisposing causes for high mortality rates. Further, frequent child-bearing and long lactational periods lead to the well known "maternal depletion" syndrome. This adversely affects women's health and aggravates, directly and indirectly, the risk of disease, disability, and death.

Maternal Morbidity and Maternal Health Care

No specific statistics or even estimates for SEAR countries are available to measure the extent of maternal morbidity, although it is well accepted that maternity-related ailments are far more frequent occurrences than maternal deaths. Small studies point to a considerable incidence of gynecological and sexually transmitted diseases. The unrelieved suffering from maternity-related problems, which range from minor to life threatening in severity, is cause for serious concern.

Steady progress in the coverage of maternal health care services has taken place. Despite the improvements, however, it remains a sad reality that in many countries of the Region very large numbers of women carry out society's most basic functions of child-bearing without the minimal support needed, such as antenatal care and trained assistance at delivery.

Only DPR Korea, Mongolia, and Sri Lanka report high coverage during childbirth by trained health personnel. In all other SEAR countries very substantial proportions of deliveries still occur without trained supervision. Thailand reports 40% of deliveries covered. In Indonesia and India only 31% and 33% of births, respectively, have trained supervision. Bhutan, Bangladesh, and Nepal have reached only between 5% and 7% coverage for delivery (Table 14-13). Tetanus toxoid protection remains in the range of 30% to 40% for pregnant women in the majority of SEAR countries. Contraceptive prevalence is around two-thirds in two countries and one-half in one. In all other countries it is far lower, ranging from 5% to 34%.

Table 14-13. Maternal Health Care in Selected South-East Asia Region Countries.

Country	Births Attended by Trained Health Personnel (%) (1983-88)	Pregnant Women Immunized Against Tetanus (%) (1987-88)	Contraceptive Prevalence Rate (1980-87)
Bangladesh	5	11	22
Bhutan	7	42	
DPR Korea	65		
India	33	58	34
Indonesia	31	33	48
Mongolia	99		
Myanmar	57	24	5
Nepal	6	31	14
Sri Lanka	87	38	62
Thailand	40	61	66

Source: State of the World's Children 1990, UNICEF.

Women's Nutrition and Anemia

Malnutrition is a widespread and major problem in the Region. It affects more numbers of persons than any other adverse condition. The World Development Report 1990 shows that per capita daily calorie supply, although improved in most SEAR countries since the mid-sixties, is still lower than the average for low income economies in four of the nine countries for which data are available (Table 14-14).

Nutritional anemia affects more than half of the women in the reproductive ages in the Region. In India, where the maximum number of maternal deaths occur, it is estimated to cause 10-20% of the maternal deaths and to affect over 60% of women. Localized surveys in Nepal report between one-half and two-thirds of women in the reproductive ages affected. The estimates of prevalence for selected SEAR countries are in Table 14-15.

Table 14-14. Daily Per Capita Calorie Supply in High and Low Income Economies and in Selected South-East Asia Region Countries; Percentage of Daily Requirements and of Low Birthweight

Country	Daily Calorie Supply Per Capita (1986)	Daily Calorie Supply as Percentage of Requirements (1984-86)	Percentage of Low Birthweight Babies (1982-88)[a]
Bangladesh	1927	83	28
DPR Korea	3232	135	
India	2238	100	30
Indonesia	2579	116	14
Mongolia	2847	116	10
Myanmar	2609	119	16
Nepal	2052	93	
Sri Lanka	2400	110	28
Thailand	2331	105	12
Countries with:			
Low Income	2384		
High Income	3376		

[a]Sri Lanka, 1981.

Sources: State of the World's Children 1990, UNICEF.
World Development Report 1990, World Bank.

Table 14-15. Prevalence of Anemia in Women of Child-bearing Age (15-49 Years) in Selected South-East Asia Region Countries

Country	Total Number of Women 15-49 Years (millions)	Women 15-49 Years Affected by Anemia	
		Number (millions)	Percentage
Bangladesh	15.9	11.0	69.2
India	139.2	84.9	61.0
Indonesia	33.0	18.6	56.4
Myanmar	7.4	3.0	40.5
Sri Lanka	3.3	2.0	60.6
Thailand	9.5	4.7	49.5

Source: Bulletin of Regional Health Informaiton 1986-87, WHO/SEARO.

POLICY SUPPORT

Women in Decision-Making

Although there have been considerable conscious efforts to increase the role of women in decision-making in the countries of the Region, this is still limited, notwithstanding the fact that top national leadership positions for some women have been easily possible in certain countries. This is evident from the numbers of women participating in public affairs. According to the indicators included in the UN WID Survey, among SEAR countries only DPR Korea and Mongolia have a substantial female presence in the countries' top legislative bodies. In Mongolia, however, which is the best-off in this regard, females account for only 25 % of the elected representatives in the legislative assembly. In DPR Korea the figure is closer to 20 %. In all other SEAR countries for which data are available, the range of female representation remains between 1 % and 11 %.

National Mechanisms and Policies

The international attention directed to the issue of women and development by the UN Decade for Women spurred the establishment of national machineries for the promotion of women's interests where none had existed and the strengthening of those already active. Among SEAR countries, Mongolia had a long-standing Committee on Women established in 1924. Eight countries (Bangladesh, Bhutan, India, Indonesia, Maldives, Nepal, Sri Lanka, and Thailand) established some type of national machinery for women's development before the end of the Women's Decade.

The mechanisms for the promotion of women's interests are in varied forms and at different levels. In three countries (Bangladesh, Indonesia, and Sri Lanka) the national machinery is at ministerial level, specifically tasked with the advancement of women. In two countries (Maldives and Thailand) the machinery is positioned directly under the leadership of the head of the executive branch, attached to the office of the Prime Minister/President. In another two countries the machinery is a part of a sectoral ministry—in India within the Ministry of Human Resource Development and in Nepal within the Ministry of Labour and Social Welfare. In two countries the responsibility rests outside government, although the National Women's Association in Bhutan works closely with the government and the National Committee on Women in Mongolia is semi-governmental.

Six of the 11 countries in the Region (Bangladesh, Bhutan, Indonesia, Mongolia, Sri Lanka, and Thailand) have ratified the United Nations Convention on the Elimination of All Forms of Discrimination Against Women (CEDAW). Two of these countries, however, have done so with reservations on certain points.

National policies for the promotion of women in development now exist in all SEAR countries. In more than half of the countries, a separate earmarked budget is also available for certain programs/projects. In several countries, separate chapters on women have been formulated in national development plans.

Legislation and Social Support

In all countries of the Region, constitutional equality of women exists. However, as the ESCAP Review of the Achievements of the Women's Decade notes, equality is not yet fully incorporated into laws on marriage and the family. The discrepancy between the statement of legal rights and the social reality is seen to be considerable. Entrenched religious or customary practices often supersede most progressive legislation which has been enacted with regard to marriage, divorce, child custody, inheritance and other civil rights in several SEAR countries. Legislation for equal pay for equal work has been enacted in a number of countries in the Region, with several countries signatories to the ILO Convention 100 on equal remuneration. But impact on the informal sector is limited.

As earlier seen, where the age of marriage is low, women are exposed to multifold dangers to health arising from early and frequent pregnancies. The role of the law in this regard remains ambivalent. In certain countries of the Region higher ages at marriage have been achieved, although the legal minimum age of marriage has continued to remain low. Examples include Sri Lanka where the legal age of marriage is 12 years for girls and 16 years for boys; Indonesia where the minimum legal age is 16 years for girls and 19 years for boys; Thailand where it is 17 years for both; and Mongolia where it is 18 years for both. In certain other countries, although a minimum age has been legislated, the actual age often remains lower, with the law being openly disregarded for traditional practices. This is the case in Bangladesh and in large parts of India, although the minimum legal age is 18 years for girls and 21 years for boys in both countries.

Drawbacks are also noted to exist in many countries with regard to other aspects of women's reproductive rights. The requirement of spousal consent to sterilization and use of contraceptives and the restriction or non-availability of legal abortion are other indicators that society formally or informally restricts women's human rights and freedoms.

Even in four of the six SEAR countries which have ratified CEDAW, some restrictions regarding sterilization procedures are noted. Abortion remains either illegal or restricted to lifesaving or abnormal sexual assault situations in four countries and available on limited grounds in a fifth. Abortion is illegal in Nepal and has only recently been made available on limited grounds in Mongolia.

Budgets for Health and Education

Strategies for cheaper and more efficient delivery of basic health care services are being actively pursued in the Region. However, the need for adequate resource allocations for health and education, particularly in the face of the enormous backlog of problems such as have been described earlier, is a key issue. Unfortunately, investments in the social development sector represented by health, education and social services continue to be modest, as reflected in Table 14-16.

Table 14-16. Central Government Expenditures Allocated (%) for Education, Health and Social Welfare for Selected South-East Asia Region Countries

Country	Education		Health		Housing, Amenities, Social Security, and Welfare	
	1972	1988	1972	1988	1972	1988
Bangladesh	14.8		5.0		9.8	
India	2.3	2.9	1.5	1.8	3.2	5.4
Indonesia	7.4	10.0	1.4	1.8	0.9	1.7
Myanmar	15.0	13.4	6.1	4.9	7.5	13.2
Nepal	7.2	10.9	4.7	4.3	0.7	3.3
Sri Lanka	13.0	7.8	6.4	5.4	19.5	11.7
Thailand	19.9	19.3	3.7	6.2	7.0	5.4

Source: World Development Report 1990, World Bank.

In 1988, the health budget in four of the six SEAR countries with available data ranged between 4.3% and 6.2% of the total expenditure, while in the case of two countries it was 1.8%. Education allocations in 1988 have fared better, ranging between 7.8% and 19.3% in five of the six reporting countries, with one country reflecting only 2.9%. It is important to note that in the six SEAR countries for which comparisons between the early seventies and late eighties are possible, expenditure on both health and education declined in two and expenditure on health alone declined in one. In two countries an increase was seen in both health and education while the sixth country showed an increase in health with a decline in education.

What clearly is important from Table 14-16 is that the allocations, particularly for health, are not commensurate with the scale of needs. As economic troubles arise, these slender budgets are being further endangered, with the effects on women, given their health situation in this Region, being particularly deleterious.

WOMEN, HEALTH AND DEVELOPMENT IN COUNTRIES OF SOUTH-EAST ASIA

WHO/SEARO promotes Women, Health, and Development (WHD) as an integrated aspect of all programme areas. The mechanisms to achieve this integration include a multi-disciplinary WHD Advisory Group with representation from various programme areas, a WHD Core Group, and focal points at country level to identify specific needs of women.

Maternal Health

Maternal health has constituted a major focus of SEARO's WHD activities. WHO has generally assisted in promoting policies and programmes emphasizing a holistic approach with integrated delivery of services. Over the last decade, considerable improvement has been made in the level of attention to maternal health, including coverage and quality of services.

Since in the majority of SEAR Member Countries more than 80% of women are delivered by traditional birth attendants (TBAs), Regional programmes have been developed with a continued focus on the training, supervision, and evaluation of TBAS. National workshops to promote TBA registration were supported in Indonesia, Nepal, and Thailand. A consultative meeting was held in December 1988 to review and revise the WHO TBA Trainers Kit. The impact of TBA training and utilization was evaluated in mid-1991 as a continuation of the above activities.

Since the International Safe Motherhood Conference in Nairobi in February 1987, most countries of the Region have implemented safe motherhood activities. National workshops have been held in Indonesia, Maldives, Nepal, and Thailand. In November 1988 eight SEAR countries participated in an intercountry workshop held on the "Safe Motherhood Initiative—Recent Developments and Key Issues."

Operational research projects directed at improving maternal health have been undertaken in many SEAR countries. These include strengthening of the maternal morbidity and mortality surveillance system in Bhutan; a multicentre control trial on the use of the partograph in Indonesia; and two studies in Nepal, one on the prevention of maternal mortality in selected hospitals and a KAP of mothers-in-law regarding maternity care of their daughters-in-law. A study on maternal mortality in Central Java, Indonesia was completed and results reviewed at a National Seminar held 1990.

Other Health and Health-Related Areas

The South-East Asia Region has actively studied the mental well-being of women and mothers, especially as related to the physical and psychological development of children (India, Sri Lanka, and Thailand). SEARO coordinated case studies on women's participation in water supply and sanitation projects with national institutions in Indonesia, Nepal, Sri Lanka, and Thailand. An intercountry workshop on the "Health Needs of Adolescents with Special Focus on Reproductive Health" was held in 1988 to focus attention on this important area.

An intercountry consultation on "Mobilization of Women's Organizations/ NGOs in the Prevention and Control of HIV Infection/AIDS" was held in May 1990. This consultation focused on critical issues concerning the implications of AIDS for women within the sociocultural context of the Region.

Future Directions

In looking forward to the future, changes that have taken place and trends established thus far, both regionally and globally, help identify general areas of priority in intensification and concentration of efforts for WHD in SEAR. Among those are areas of critical importance to women, where progress which has been achieved so far still falls short of minimally desirable standards, for example safe motherhood, nutrition, and family planning.

There is also an urgent need to obtain essential, sensitive, and country-specific information, especially gender specific, disaggregated information. Documentation of such information for sub-groups, particularly identified disadvantaged and vulnerable groups, is a prerequisite for the formulation of realistic plans of action for country level activities.

A general shifting of the locale of action to the countries and preferably the grassroots level is essential. Countries are where the action ought to be, more so now than ever. Country-specific situations where little or no data are available should become the special focus of exploration and action. Proactive and dynamic efforts to foster and support country level efforts and organizations should take precedence in the formulation of plans and activities.

Women, Health, and Development in SEAR countries need sustained and redoubled efforts so that women of the next millenium will be in a position to take their rightful place in the process of human development. Practical and sustained actions at policy and program levels covering social, economic, and political dimensions will be essential in the coming decade and the 21st century.[8]

---

[8]This report has been summarized from a draft publication titled "Women, Health and Development: South-East Asia Region." The referenced publication is an update of the 1985 WHO/SEARO Regional Health Paper No. 8 and is expected to be available by June 1992.

Western Pacific

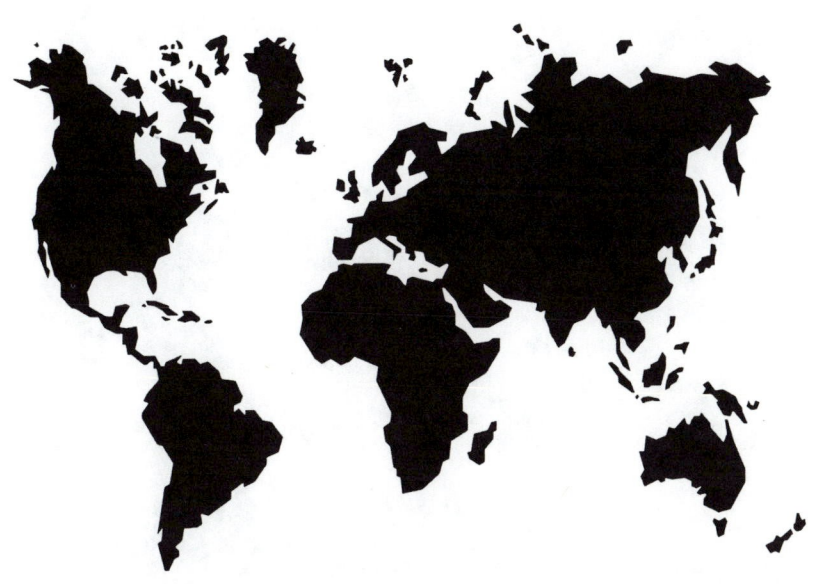

Australia
Japan
Republic of Korea

Women's Health Status in Australia

WHO Collaborating Centre For Nursing Development
in Primary Health Care
The University of Sydney
Faculty of Health Sciences

Faith M. Jones

SYNOPSIS OF COUNTRY

Area and Population

Australia comprises a land area of 7,682,300 square kilometers. The population in Australia at June 1990 was 17,086,197 persons. Table 15-1 presents the distribution of the Australian population by sex and age group.

Scheme of Parliamentary Government

Under the Australian Constitution the legislative power of the Commonwealth of Australia is vested in the parliament of the Commonwealth, which consists of the Queen, the Senate, and the House of Representatives. The Federal government is presently held by the Australian Labour Party.

Table 15-1. Australian Female Population By Age Group

Age Group (years)	Population	%
0-9	1,225,573	14.3
10-19	1,284,415	15.0
20-29	1,368,840	16.0
30-39	1,351,466	15.7
40-49	1,102,295	12.8
50-59	758,096	8.8
60-69	719,879	8.4
70-79	493,913	5.7
80-84	141,394	1.6
85+	109,123	1.2
Total	8,554,994	100.0

Source: ABS Australian Demographic Statistics June Quarter 1990. (3101.0).
Note. Total male population = 8,531,203.

Ethnic Divisions and Languages

Australia today is a multi-ethnic society (Table 15-2). The aboriginal people of Australia remain an important ethnic group. Australia also contains many people from parts of Europe, and a growing number of people from East Asia and Southeast Asia.

This ethnic diversity is accompanied by linguistic diversity. Over 2 million people aged 5 years and over (14%), spoke a language other than English at home (Table 15-3). This has a major impact on the educational and health care system. Many women and their families need translation services in order to communicate appropriately with their health care providers.

EDUCATION/LITERACY

Literacy Rates

A survey of adult literacy skills in 1990 revealed that 10% of adults over the age of 18 years have low levels of literacy within Australia. Those with a low literacy include 72% of English speaking born compared to 28% of non-English speaking adults. The survey showed no gender differences. Persons over 55 years old and persons with less than 6 years of schooling were most likely to have low literacy performance. (*Source:* Institute of Technical & Adult Teacher Education. *A Survey of Australian Adult Literacy 1990.* Author Rose Wickert.)

Table 15-2. Ethnic Classification of Australian Population

Ancestry	Numbers (1,000)
English	5,561.6
Australasian	2,905.8
Italian	507.2
Irish	337.6
Scottish	339.8
Greek	293.0
British so described	285.1
English-Irish	258.8
German	233.3
Australian-English	194.3
English-Scottish	183.0
Chinese	172.5
Aboriginal	153.0
Dutch	149.7
English-German	115.9
Yugoslavian	109.5
Polish	97.1
Maltese	96.8
Irish-Scottish	88.6
Lebanese	82.4
Vietnamese	62.2
Indian	46.7
Welsh	45.5
Other Britain	45.2
New Zealand	44.5
Spanish	43.1
Other not classifiable	2,043.2
Not stated	1,066.5
Total	15,602.1

Source: ABS *Multicultural Australia 1990.* (2505.0).

Schools

Proportionally more girls than boys have stayed in school until year 12. While the retention rate for boys and girls has increased in recent years, the gender gap in the retention rate has also increased (Table 15-4).

Table 15-3. Non-English Languages Spoken in Australia

Language	%
Italian	3.0
Greek	1.9
Yugoslavian	1.0
Chinese	0.9
German	0.8
Arabic/Lebanese	0.7
Spanish	0.5
Polish	0.5
Dutch	0.4
Vietnamese	0.4
Maltese	0.4
French	0.4
Total Percent	14.0

Source: ABS Multicultural Australia 1990. (2505.0).
Total Number = 2,022,800.

Table 15-4. Education Retention Rates to Year 12

Year	Female (%)	Male (%)	GEI(Female/Male)
1987	57.0	49.4	1.15
1988	61.8	53.4	1.16
1989	65.2	55.5	1.17
1990	69.9	58.3	1.20

Source: ABS Schools Australia. (4221.0)

Higher Education

The higher education of women continues to improve as the female share of total higher education students has increased from 48.8% in 1986 to 52.7% in 1990. Growth in female enrollments has continued to outpace that of males, so that the female share of total enrollments rose to 53% in 1990. Of the total female students enrolled in 1990 (255,655), 84.1% (215,074) were undergraduates and 4.3% master's and 1.3% PhD or higher. The total number of males registered in higher education programs was 229,420, for a female/male ratio of 1.1/1.0.

Arts and education continue to dominate female enrollments, although their share of total female enrollments has fallen from 72% in 1979 to 50% in 1990. In 1990, female students accounted for around 70% of education, health and arts students, but only 10% of engineering students. However, females' share of engineering enrollments has risen over previous years (Table 15-5). Women's share of postgraduate enrollments is lower than their share of undergraduate enrollments, in all broad fields of study.

Table 15-5. Women in Higher Education by Field of Study

Field of Study	%
Agriculture	1.1
Architecture	1.4
Arts	29.1
Business	16.7
Education	21.2
Engineering	1.4
Health	15.4
Law	2.5
Science	10.2
Veterinary Science	0.3
Non-award	0.7
Total	100.0

Total Number = 255,655.

HEALTH CARE

Australian Health Care System

Australia provides both a public and private health care system. It has adopted a Primary Health Care model, as designated by the World Health Organization's Health For All by the Year 2000 initiative.

Major Health Concerns

In March 1987 the Australian Health Ministers' Advisory Council established the Health Targets and Implementation (Health for All) Committee to develop a set of health goals and targets for Australia for the year 2000. Goals (and where appropriate, targets) have been set in three major areas: population groups, major causes of illness and death, and risk factors.

Health Goals and Targets, 1987

1. Population groups:
   -Aborigines
   -Migrants
   -Women
   -Men
   -Older people
   -Children
   -Adolescents
   -Socioeconomically disadvantaged

2. Major causes of sickness and death:
   -Heart disease
   -Stroke
   -Cancers; lung cancer, breast cancer, cervical cancer, skin cancer
   -Injury
   -Musculoskeletal diseases
   -Diabetes
   -Disability
   -Dental disease
   -Mental illness
   -Asthma

3. Risk factors:
   -Drugs, including tobacco smoking, alcohol misuse, pharmaceutical misuse or abuse, illicit drugs, and substance abuse
   -Nutrition
   -Physical inactivity
   -High blood pressure
   -High blood cholesterol
   -Occupational heath hazards
   -Unprotected sexual activity
   -Environmental heath hazards

(Source: Health For All Australians: Report of the Health Targets and Implementation [Health for All] Committee to Australian Health Ministers 1988.)

Health Demographic

Life Expectancy. Women in Australia, like women in most other industrialized countries, can expect to live substantially longer than men. Australian men currently have a life expectancy of 73.9 years at birth, while the life expectancy at birth for women is 80.0 years. Males at 65 years have an average life expectancy of 80.2 years, while women at 65 years have a life expectancy of 84.0 years. (*Source:* ABS *Deaths Australia 1990.* [3302.0])

Death Rates. There were 120,062 deaths registered in Australia, with 64,660 males and 55,402 females. The crude death rate decreased to 7.0 per 1000 population from 7.4 in 1989. The median age at death was 71.9 for males and 78.7 for females.

Infant Mortality. Perinatal death statistics include only foetuses and infants weighing at least 500 grams. In 1990 there were 2,712 perinatal deaths, of which 1,590 were foetal deaths and 1,122 were neonatal deaths. The perinatal death rate was 10.3 deaths per 1000 births; 1,087 foetal deaths occurred before labour commenced. Fifty-two percent occurred within 1 day to less than 7 days prior to commencement of labour.

The perinatal mortality rate was higher for males than females overall and for both foetal and neonatal deaths. The sex ratio of perinatal deaths was 133 males per 100 males. The sex ratio was 126:100 for foetal deaths and 148:100 for neonatal deaths. (*Source:* ABS *Perinatal Deaths Australia 1990.* [3304.0])

Women's Health. Three out of four women in the age group 15-44 years had received an injection against Rubella. Over 90% of those in the 15-24 years age group bracket had been vaccinated. One out of five of those who had not been vaccinated reported that they had never bothered or not thought about it.

Three out of four of the women aged 18-50 years had a child or children (less than 5 years) at the time of the survey and reported breastfeeding one or more of these children. Of those children aged 18 months to 5 years who were breast fed, over half had breast fed for periods of more than 6 months.

Preliminary findings show that 85% of women aged 18-64 years reported having a Pap smear test for evidence of cervical cancer, at some time. Of these women, half had been tested within the past year. Approximately 12% of women in this age group reported having had a hysterectomy.

Most women (70%) said that they had at some time had a doctor or medical assistant conduct a breast examination for signs of cancer. Almost two out of three said that they regularly conduct breast self-examinations. About one in three women reported having had a mammogram. (*Source:* ABS *National Heath Survey: Preliminary Statistics Australia 1989-90.* [4361.0])

Children's Immunization. Approximately 95% of children aged 6 years or less have had a Triple Antigen (TA) or combined Diphtheria and Tetanus (CDT) injection. Preliminary findings show that about 92% of children (under 6 years) have been vaccinated against mumps, and six out of seven against measles.

Health Care System/Financing: 1991 Budget Highlights

Budget Priorities

1. Early Detection of Cervical Cancer was funded for $22.4 million over 4 years. New directions in screening for cervical cancer will be promoted, including an information campaign, improving the reliability of Pap smears, a program of education for service providers and funding for the States and Territories for infrastructure.

2. National Women's Health Program was funded for $28.0 million over 2 years. Funding projects to improve health services for women, particularly for those who suffer access to health care; information and education schemes to inform women on health issues; and training and education on women's health issues for heath care professionals. (*Source:* Office of the Status of Women, Dept. of the Prime Minister & Cabinet, *National Agenda for Women: Implementation Report 1991.*)

ECONOMICS

Income

The average weekly earnings of all employees in August 1991 was $575 for males and $384 for females. (ABS *Monthly Summary of Statistics Australia January 1992* [1304.0].)

Labour Force Participation

Women in occupations by major groupings are presented in Table 15-6. The number of persons in varied health occupations is presented in Table 15-7. Registered nurses represent 54% of the work force in health occupations.

One Parent Families

In Australia, 14.9% of all families with dependent children are single parent families, with 85.7% of these headed by women as compared to 14.3% of all families headed by men (Table 15-8).

Table 15-6. Occupations of Employed Persons, November 1991

Occupational Group	Total Group Work Force (1,000)	Fe-male%
Managers and Administrators	885.1	26.2
Professionals	1,003.3	41.3
Paraprofessional	471.8	46.3
Tradespersons	1,154.9	10.0
Clerks	1,293.9	72.1
Sales Persons and Personal Service Work-ers	1,155.3	64.4
	555.7	16.5
Plant and Machine Operators and Drivers	1,154.2	35.2
Labourers and Related Workers		
Total Workforce	7,674.1	42.0

Source: ABS *Monthly Summary of Statistics Australia January 1992.* (1304.0)

Table 15-7. Persons Employed In Health Occupations, 1986

Health Occupations	Number
Gen. Medical Practitioner	23,790
Spec. Medical Practitioner	9,000
Dental Practitioner	6,310
Pharmacists	10,640
Occup. Therapists	2,770
Optometrists	1,470
Physiotherapists	5,930
Speech Pathologists	1,320
Chiropractors and Osteopaths	1,370
Podiatrists	980
Radiographers	4,270
Other health diagnosis and treatment practitioners	4,659
Registered Nurses	138,220
Enrolled Nurses	35,220
Dental Nurses	8,800
Total	253,970

Source: ABS Characteristics of Persons Employed in Health Occupations, Australia 1989. (4346.0).

Table 15-8. Female Labour Force Participation Rates In Single Parent Families

Labor Force Statistics	Mothers (%)
In Labour Force	42.4
Employed	34.8
Unemployed	7.6
Not In Labour Force	57.6

Source: ABS Australia's One Parent Families: Census, 1986 (2511.0).

FAMILY STRUCTURE

Marital Status

In 116,959 marriages in Australia in 1990, 39.8% of husbands were over 30 years of age compared with 28.9% of wives. The median age at marriage was 28.1 years for males and 25.8 years for females. The median age for those who were married for the first time was 26.4 years for males and 24.3 years for females. The median age for marriages of divorced persons was 39.5 years for males and 36.0 for females. In 1990, 42,635 people were divorced. In this group the median age for males was 38.2 years and 35.3 years for females. (*Sources:* ABS *Marriages Australia 1991* [3306.0] and ABS *Divorce Australia 1991* [3307.0])

Division of Property and Rights of Children upon Divorce

The Family Law Act 1975 commenced operation on January 5, 1976, and stipulates that there is only one grounds for divorce—that of irretrievable breakdown of a marriage. These grounds are established when the husband and wife have been separated and have lived apart from each other for 12 months and there is no reasonable likelihood of their reconciliation. Provisions of the Family Law Act dealing with the maintenance, custody, and welfare of children of a marriage have, since April 1, 1988, applied to all children (including ex-nuptial children) in New South Wales, Victoria, South Australia, Tasmania, the Australian Capital Territory, and Norfolk Island. In Queensland and in Western Australia, the Family Law Act does not apply to ex-nuptial children, who are subject to state laws.

In relation to the guardianship and custody of children, the Family Law Act provides that both parents and guardians, subject to a court order to the contrary, have joint custody of children under the age of 18. However, a parent or another interested person can apply to the court for sole custody of a child at any time.

In disputes in which the welfare of a child is in issue, a child may be separately represented. The paramount consideration for the court in the determination of all such disputes is the welfare of the child. A court is guided by statutory considerations, which include, where appropriate, the wishes of the child. Parents of a child may agree on custody and guardianship matters and register their agreement in a court. In relation to the welfare of children, a divorce decree usually will not become effective unless the Court is satisfied that proper arrangements have been made by the parties for the welfare of their children.

There are certain specific matters for the Court to consider when it is dealing with maintenance applications. These include:

* the age and state of health of the parties;

* the income, property and financial resources of each of the parties and their financial obligations;

* the length of the marriage and what is an appropriate standard of living for each party;

* whether either party has to care for children;

* the extent to which the marriage has effected the earning capacity of the applicant; and

* the possibility of the applicant taking on a training course or further educational course to improve his or her employment perspectives.

The act also provides for the registration of, and court approval for, maintenance agreements made by the parties. The Court has power to settle disputes about the parties' family assets, including the power to order a transfer of legal interests in property. When dealing with these disputes, the Court considers the interest each party has in the property, the financial and non-financial contributions made by each party during the marriage, and matters the Court is required to consider in dealing with maintenance applications. (*Source:* ABS *Australian Year Book 1991*. [3101.0])

POLITICAL PARTICIPATION OF WOMEN

Voting Rights

All Australian citizens who are at least 18 years of age and possess certain residential qualifications are required to vote for members of the Parliaments of each state. For the Commonwealth Parliament the qualifications for the franchise are identical for both houses, extending to Australian citizens and British subjects who are on the Commonwealth Electoral Roll and who are not less than 18 years of age.

Women in Political Positions

In July 1991, the percentage of women in the Federal Parliament was 12.5% (comprising 23.7% of the Senate and 6.8% of the House of Representatives). Women represent 13.4% of all State and Territory Parliamentarians, although in some cases the figure was considerably higher—for example, women currently comprise 35.6% of the New South Wales Legislative Council and 22.7% of the South Australian Legislative Council. There are currently three women amongst the eight Premiers and Chief Ministers. (*Source:* Office Of The Status of Women, Department of the Prime Minister & Cabinet *National Agenda For Women; Implementation Report 1991.*)

NATIONAL AGENDA FOR WOMEN

The National Agenda for Women is an annual publication published by the Office of the Status of Women. It is a key element of the Government's ongoing commitment to equality of opportunity in Australian society, in particular its commitment to ensuring that Australian women enjoy a say, a choice, and a fair go.

The Government has adopted the objectives of the National Agenda for Women as the focus for the development and implementation of its strategy for women. As well, the Government adopted the following 20 action plans for implementation in the five years from 1988 to 1992.

1. Consultation and participation in decision making
2. Education
3. Women at home
4. Employment and training
5. Child care
6. Leisure
7. Care for older women
8. Sex discrimination
9. Portrayal of women in the media
10. Income security
11. Superannuation
12. Housing
13. Violence against women and children
14. Health
15. Aboriginal and Torres Strait Islander Women
16. Immigrant and NESB Women

17. Women and disabilities
18. Young women
19. Women living in rural and regional areas, and
20. International cooperation

(*Source:* Office Of The Status of Women, Department of the Prime Minister & Cabinet *National Agenda for Women: Implementation Report 1991.*)

DISCUSSION

For a country as large as Australia, with vast areas of desert, scrubland, dividing ranges and surrounded by beaches, it is not surprising that the population is quite sparse. In the eastern, southern, and south western seaboards, the population has an older female population, i.e., from 60 to 85+ years of age with a large male population in all other age groups except those between 35 to 39 years of age.

In such a country that is so heavily populated by males it is apparent that when the Australian Health Ministers Advisory Council established the Health Targets & Implementation (Health For All) Committee in 1987, women were listed as a group in and of themselves. However, within the socioeconomically disadvantaged, the Aboriginal, adolescents, older people, or migrants, which were also listed as separate groups, women also would be included.

Of the diseases that affect the population generally, heart disease, stroke and cancers are the major causes of sickness and death. Drug abuse, including tobacco and alcohol, is the leading risk factor, with poor nutrition and physical inactivity following close behind.

These statistics are taken for the total population. While pockets of poverty can be seen both in rural and urban areas, Australia has prided itself on the active lifestyle of its people and the abundance of nutritious fruit, vegetables, fish, and meat that are readily available. However, the country also has had a history of excessive drinking, and until recently, smoking tobacco was considered a way of life for old and young. For women, these diseases and risk factors are just as threatening as for men. Although women live longer on the average of 4-7 years more than their male colleagues, the diseases have similar rates for both sexes.

The Australian health care system has had a rigorous tradition of being able to treat all who needed care. The public health care was efficient and provided assistance from birth to the grave. For those wishing it, a small private health care system was also available. With over 250,000 health workers for a population of 8 million, the ratio of health workers to the people appears to be adequate.

However, as there are pockets of poverty, the health care system also has groups of people who are not receiving adequate health care. People in the rural sector, Aboriginals and migrants, often are not able to access the system.

Adopting an "Australian Health For All" scheme, a network of community centers were developed to meet the needs of the elderly, babies and young children and the mentally ill.

Unfortunately, the huge influx of migrants into the country in the 1980s and 1990s inundated services. The inability to speak English and to understand the instructions of getting to a Center has been an important reason that the Department of Health in New South Wales, for example, print information in as many as 120 languages.

Special programs for women have been established by individual States to improve services and to give information concerning children and women's health. Immunization campaigns have reiterated the need for prevention of infectious diseases. Educational programs to encourage breastfeeding has had an important effect on the numbers of women continuing breastfeeding—some until the baby is 6 months of age.

There is a strong trend in Australia for the "de facto" marriage. This is a legal status. As well, the number of one parent families has escalated since 1986. Lone single mothers make up 85.7% of all single parents. The statistics concerning the opportunity and ability to work is half that of lone single fathers. Thus, for women, the future opportunities for advancement are limited. However, more women are able to enter higher education programs and, currently, over half the students in universities are women.

The Office of the Status of Women has planned for an improvement in women's health, education and welfare by the Year 2000. The *National Agenda for Women* detailed various issues that must be dealt with by the end of the decade. However, 20 of those issues were targeted to be accomplished by 1992. The health of women was prioritized as Number 14, behind such problems as education, child care, care for older women, and income security. The Australian Government has accomplished much to improve women's health in the 1990s. It is now trying to improve the quality of life for specific groups of women. The thousands of migrants who arrive in Australia each year are particularly hard pressed to access the health service. Aboriginals have a difficult time in accessing the health system as villages in the rural outback are situated thousands of miles from hospitals or health centers.

The Australian Government needs to work with the women of these specific groups to ascertain their needs for better health care. The top priority of the *National Agenda for Women* was that the government was to consult with women and participate with them in decision making. Slowly, this objective is being met—especially as Australian women become more politically able to lobby for better health care.

16

Women's Health Status in Japan

World Health Organization
Collaborating Centre For Nursing Development
In Primary Health Care
St. Luke's College of Nursing, Tokyo, Japan

Choko Arai and Yasuko Mitsuhashi

COUNTRY AND GENERAL DEMOGRAPHICS

The Japanese archipelago includes four main islands that make up only 0.3% of the land portion of the earth's surface. The total land area is slightly less than that of the U.S. state of California or the European nation of Sweden. Mountainous areas cover 70% of the nation. Much of the land that was once rich agricultural land is now being used for buildings, highways, and commercial purposes. After excluding areas unsuitable for living, the Japanese population density is the highest in the world. The 1990 census indicated a population of 123,612,000, 3% of the earth's population. Despite the population density, the limited amount of available land, and the many typhoons and earthquakes that strike Japan, it is unique in Asia as a major, fully industrialized, capitalistic economic power. The Japanese enjoy close to 100% literacy rate. Japanese is the language of the people although English is taught from junior high school. Japan is a predominantly homogenous Mongoloid country, a fact that limits internalization of the society. There is a democratic form of government.

Health Concerns and Health Demographics

The economic and technological successes of Japan do not exempt it from major health concerns. At present 12% of the population is aged 65 or older and is expected to increase to 25% by 2020. Increase in the aging population is accompanied by the requirement for a new complex health care delivery system and the means to support it. Life expectancy for women is age 81.81 and for men is 75.86. This increases the number of frail elderly, particularly frail elderly women. Longer life also increases the rate of chronic illness and the need for specialized health and medical information and services.

Advances in health science information present the challenge of health information dissemination to the entire population. Issues such as the right to choice of treatment, the right to know details of treatment, informed consent, and self-determination are complicated by large numbers of persons processed through a strained health care delivery system. These problems are complicated further when the clients are aged. Elderly clients often retain older cultural customs and expectations within a busy modern system. Older cultural customs defined the place of women in society much differently than presently defined.

Rapid increase in the use of high technology and professionalization of health care workers presents the challenge of achieving and maintaining health care laborers. Greater technology requires more trained laborers and greater professionalization requires longer schooling. Both will delay preparation of needed numbers of health care professionals. Further, the 1990 birth rate was 9.9/1000 and the death rate was 6.7/1000. Currently, not only is there a great shortage of health care professionals, but there will simply not be enough people to enter health care professions in the future. Women, a traditional source of low cost and undemanding labor, are less willing to accept jobs at the bottom of the system. Even if there were enough workers, the question of financial capacity would arise. Table 16-1 shows the population pyramid and the number of males per 100 females in each age group.

Increases in technology and knowledge do not come without a cost. Japan is now asking who will create the capital to bear the burden of the quantity and quality of health care expenses. Women are increasingly entering the work force out of the home. Questions of benefits versus cost and efficiency of the medical care system are coming into focus as never before.

Ethical questions involve not only economics but dilemmas regarding life and death issues. Japan has not yet defined death as brain death, a problem particularly affecting those who seek transplantation and other sophisticated care. Care of terminally ill persons and death with dignity are issues being addressed. Reproductive issues are also being questioned. Women's control over their own bodies and reproductive rights are being examined. Birth using the technologies of frozen sperm, in vitro fertilization, fetal diagnosis and surgery, and genetic engineering related to hereditary diseases are sources of great concern and debate.

Table 16-1. Number and Ratio of Males to 100 Females in Each Age Category

Age	Number (1,000s)	Ratio of Males to Females
0-4	6,698	105.460
5-9	7,559	104.962
10-14	8,805	105.149
15-19	9,963	105.295
20-24	8,729	104.179
25-29	7,845	102.922
30-34	7,835	101.776
35-39	9,466	101.083
40-44	10,011	100.661
45-49	9,175	98.894
50-54	8,018	97.902
55-59	7,558	91.126
60-64	6,548	96.209
65-69	4,874	72.530
70-74	3,648	70.387
75-79	2,938	66.045
80-84	1,725	59.426
85-89	797	49.812
90+	269	39.378
Total	122,460	96.599

In this densely populated, increasingly expensive, primarily older society there is a health care system frantically trying to keep pace. Within the society as well as the health care system there are issues of women's health and development that beg for solutions.

THE HEALTH CARE SYSTEM, FINANCING, AND UTILIZATION

Health Care Delivery System

The total national medical care expenditure in Japan must be put into the context of the nationally supported health insurance plans and the public health center system. Everyone in Japan is covered by some type of health insurance although there are no private health insurance plans. The Employee's Health Insurance covers six categories of workers. Health Insurance Societies of Mutual Aid Associations finance, and where these do not exist, the national government does it. Anyone who does not come under the six categories of workers will come under the National Health Insurance (NHI) program which is financed by national and local governments and public interest groups. Disability allowance, nursing allowance, maternity allowance, and funeral expenses are covered on a case by case basis. Low income households or specific chronic disease cases are granted additional subsidies by the government. Health insurance for the aged is included in the NHI program.

In 1989 the Japanese national medical care expenditure (NME) was 19,729 thousand million yen (US $157 billion). This is 160,100 yen (US $1,280) per capita. The proportion of the NME was 4.86% of the Gross National Product. The NME in 1989 is itemized on Table 16-2. Personal out-of-pocket expenses were 12.3% of the total expenditures. Hospitals and clinics receive direct pay from the insurance programs and the remaining co-payment is paid out of pocket by the client at the time of care. Families are registered by the employment of the head of the household, usually the father's employer. On the National Health Insurance plan anyone may register at the city office where they reside and pay monthly premiums based on their monthly income. The out-of-pocket expenses for the client vary with each of these plans. Health coverage also includes funeral coverage.

The goals of Public Health Centers (PHC) are the promotion of environmental health and the prevention of disease. They coordinate all community health programs for maternal and child health, adult health guidance and rehabilitation, inspection and control of environmental sanitation, infectious disease control, and statistics of all kinds.

In 1989 a proposal was made to establish a health center for every secondary health care district. The regional medical care plan was expanded to include education of residents of the city town or village. The major goals of public health centers are to 1) spread the concept of health; 2) keep health and welfare statistics; 3) improve nutrition and sanitation of food; 4) monitor home environmental health; 5) provide public health nurses; 6) improve public medical care facilities; 7) monitor the health of expectant mothers, children, and the aged; 8) promote dental hygiene; 9) provide physical examinations; 10) promote mental health; and 11) prevent illness, particularly tuberculosis, sexually transmitted diseases, and infections.

The goals of the city health centers are similar to the public centers but provide comprehensive services. These include counseling, health education, and physical examinations. Because it is close to home this service is meant to be efficient and respond to the felt needs of the residents. Providers respond to the expressed needs of the recipients providing increased autonomy and self control. The number of centers proposed is 1,106. An increased number of locations providing access to health care also means an increased number of health care providers to staff the locations. Table 16-3 shows the 1990 data on the categories

Table 16-2. Percentage of National Medical Care Expenditures in 1989

Type of Expenditure	%
A. Public Expense Total	5.6
Daily Life Security Law	3.8
Tuberculosis Control Law	0.2
Mental Health Law	0.4
Others	1.2
B. Social Insurance Total	54.7
Employee's Health Insurance	
Government Managed Health Insurance	15.5
Society Managed Health Insurance	11.5
Seaman's Insurance	0.2
National Civil Service Mutual Aid Association	1.5
Local Civil Service Mutual Aid Association	2.9
Private School Teachers and Employees Mutual Aid Association	0.3
National Health Insurance	21.0
Others	1.7
C. Medical Service for the Aged	
	27.4
D. Personal Expense	
	13.3

of health workers, the total numbers, and the average number per 100,000 population. The nurses of all kinds account for the largest numbers and the total largest percentage of all health care providers.

Health Service Utilization

There were 1,287,302 reported pregnancies in 1989. Table 16-4 indicates the number of women who received health instruction including physical examination in 1989. Table 16-5 indicates that babies are born primarily in hospitals. There are high rates of infant immunizations. Mothers see this as a duty of motherhood. Also, great care is taken in the preschool to assure compliance.

Table 16-3. Total Number and Average Rate per 100,000 of Health Workers at Medical Institutions or Pharmacies, 1988

Category of Worker	Number	Rate per 100,000
Physicians	193,682	157.7
Dentists	68,692	55.9
Pharmacists	84,302	68.7
Public health nurses	25,303	20.5
Midwives	22,918	18.5
Nurses and Assistant Nurses	745,301	602.9
Dental hygienists	40,932	33.1
Dental technicians	32,433	26.2
Anna-massager and Fingure pressure therapist	91,969	74.4
Needle therapist and Cauterize therapist	119,960	97.0
Judo-seihuku-shi	22,904	18.8

Table 16-4. Women Receiving Instruction and Number of Problems Detected

Condition	Total	At PHC	At City
Pregnant Women			
Receiving first health instruction	504,800	174,285	330,515
Detection of edema, proteinuria, hypertension	9,621	3,547	6,074
Detection of other pregnancy problems	39,313	18,448	20,865
Expectant Mothers			
Receiving first health instruction	356,923	245,335	111,568
Detection of problems	18,753	12,424	6,328
Others			
Receiving first health instruction	233,515	69,57	163,938
Detection of problems	43,679	20,699	22,980

Table 16-5. Where Babies Are Born

Year	Hospitalized (Hospital, Clinic, Midwife Clinic)			Nonhospital (Home, etc.) Total
	Total	Urban Area	Rural Area	
1950	4.6	11.3	1.1	95.4
1955	17.6	28.2	6.6	82.4
1960	50.1	63.3	27.0	49.9
1965	84.0	90.3	67.8	16.0
1970	96.1	97.6	91.2	3.9
1975	98.8	99.2	97.4	1.2
1980	99.5	99.7	99.1	0.5
1985	99.8	99.8	99.6	0.2
1989	99.9	99.9	99.8	0.1

EDUCATION, ECONOMICS AND FAMILY STRUCTURE

Educational Achievement of Women

Japan requires education for both boys and girls from age 7 through 15. Education for both men and women has steadily increased since 1955. However, the disparity between men and women has widened rather than narrowed over time. Admission to high school, junior college, college, and higher education becomes less equally distributed between men and women as the years go on. The rate of admission of women to college and higher degree programs lags considerably behind that of men (Table 16-6). Admission rates tell only part of the story. Table 16-7 indicates the number of female graduates in advanced degrees and the ratio of male to female from 1990 data. Clearly, women in Japan do not attain levels of education as high as men.

Employment and Economics of Women

The differences among average monthly per capita income in 1990 can be demonstrated by indicating persons who are employed in large and small companies. Companies that have over 30 employees give their workers ¥370,169 (US $2,961) per month and those companies that have 5 or fewer employees give their workers ¥329,443 (US $2,635.) per month. These figures include tax, premiums for social insurance, etc.

Table 16-6. Admission to School Beyond Age 15, by Gender

Year	Total	Male	Female	Total	Male	Female
		High School			Junior College	
1955	51.5	55.5	47.4	2.2	1.9	2.6
1960	57.7	59.6	55.9	2.1	1.2	3
1965	70.7	71.7	69.6	4.1	1.7	6.7
1970	82.1	81.6	82.7	6.5	2	11.2
1975	91.9	91	93	11	2.6	19.9
1980	94.2	93.1	95.4	11.3	2	21
1985	93.8	92.8	94.9	11.1	2	20.8
1986	93.8	92.8	94.9	11.1	1.8	21
1987	93.9	92.8	95	11.4	1.8	20.5
1988	94.1	92.9	95.3	11.6	1.8	21.8
1989	94.1	93	95.3	11.7	1.7	22.1
1990	94.4	93.2	95.6	11.7	1.7	22.2
1991	94.6	95.8	93.5	12.2	1.8	23.1
	College and University			Master's and Doctor's Degree		
1955	7.9	13.1	2.4			
1960	8.2	13.7	2.5	4.2	4.7	1.9
1965	12.8	20.7	4.6	4.4	5.1	1.5
1970	17.1	27.3	6.5	4.3	5.1	1.7
1975	26.7	40.4	12.5	3.9	4.7	1.6
1980	26.1	39.3	12.3	5.5	6.5	2.5
1985	26.5	38.6	13.7	5.7	6.7	2.8
1986	23.6	34.2	12.5	6	7.1	2.9
1987	24.7	35.3	13.6	6.1	7.3	2.7
1988	25.1	35.3	14.4	6.3	7.6	3
1989	24.7	34.1	14.7	6.4	7.7	3.1
1990	24.6	33.4	15.2			
1991	25.5	34.5	16.1			

Table 16-7. Graduates with Advanced Degrees

Degree	Total	Male	Female
Master's	25,804	22,226	3,578
Doctorate	5,812	5,116	696

Other inequalities exist. Households of the elderly and fatherless households (with only mother and children) have about half the income of other households of equal numbers. These people are not increasing their income at the same pace as others in the society . During a 5-year period income of all households in Japan increased by an average of ¥690,000 (US $5,520). Fatherless households had an increase of only ¥20,000 (US $160) during the same 5-year period. Only part of the fatherless households are secured by the Daily Life Security Law. The amount of security of a fatherless household was ¥158,848 (US $1,270) per month which is ¥1,901,182 (US $15,209) per year. This is barely the minimum standard of living for women. Table 16-8 presents data on the type of households and income differentials.

Table 16-8. Percentage of Types of Households and Income Differential

Household Type	Percentage	Average Annual Income	Per Capita
Total	100.0		
Elderly	10.4	5,667,000	1,746,000
Mother and child	1.3	2,750,000	1,770,000
Father and child	0.3	2,271,000	942,000
Others	88.0	6,114,000	1,754,000

Of households in Japan, 8.2% are covered by the Daily Life Security Law. Of these households, 11.7% are mother-child households. About four-fifths of the households are elderly, handicapped, or ill..

As of 1990 women comprise 40.6% of the labor force in Japan. The comparison between working aged men and women by labor indicates that traditional roles related to household work continue (Table 16-9).

Women in the work force have been increasing with the decline in the birth rate. The pattern of women working forms a unique M curve. There is a rise in numbers of women at work during age 25-29 with a sharp slump following. Then again after age 30-34 there is a marked upward trend. Women return to work after their children have begun school.

The jobs that men and women engage in form a sharp contrast that can be seen on Table 16-10. Many women select part time work and far fewer are executives. However, in general there have been improvements in the equal treatment of women and men in the work place. Women in skilled labor and engineering are increasing.

Table 16-9. Type of Daily Activity of the Working Aged Population

Characteristic	Female	Male
Total over age 15 in the population	1,780,000	49,110,000
Total labor force participation	25,930,000	37,130,000
Percent of the population working	50.1	77.2
Working		
Self-employed	10.5	16.0
Household work	16.4	42.5
Employee	70.7	79.2
Agriculture		
Self-employed	18.1	77.2
Household work	77.0	14.6
Employee	5.4	8.7
Unemployed	2.2	2.0
Percent of the population not working	49.5	22.3
Household work	59.1	
Student	17.6	
Other	23.3	

Table 16-10. Percentage of Men and Women in Selected Jobs

Job	Female	Male
Manager of a private business	3.6	8.5
Regular employee	60.6	83.2
Part time (5+ hours daily)	26.3	0.7
Fill in part time (few days/week)	5.5	3.3
Temporary	0.3	0.1
Commission earners	1.5	1.6
Other	2.2	2.5

In 1986 the Equal Employment Opportunity Law was enacted. Since that time many companies needing new employees no longer specify gender when they hire. Article 8 of this law calls for equality in promotion and job assignment. There has not been strict adherence to this Article to date. However, women are accepted into many occupations that have never before been available.

Table 16-11 shows the ratio of women in various kinds of occupations. Perhaps the largest discrepancy is in managerial positions.

Table 16-11. Occupations by Female and Male Percentages, 1990

Occupation	Percentage of Structure		Ratio of Women in Employees
	Female	Male	
Total	100.0	100.0	37.9
Professional or technical occupations	13.8	11.3	42.6
Managerial occupations	1.0	7.2	7.7
Office work	34.4	16.2	58.0
Sales	12.5	15.0	33.8
Agriculture, Forestry, Fishery	0.6	0.9	28.2
Mining worker	0.0	0.1	0.0
Transportation, Correspondence	0.5	6.9	4.2
Engineer, Operator of production process	20.6	32.2	28.2
Laborer	5.6	4.8	41.6
Prevention of peace (or safety), Service	10.7	6.2	51.3

Family Structure

With the entry of more women into the labor force there have been dramatic changes in the traditional family structure and function. Modern marriage practices have gone far ahead of the older laws that are still in force related to family structure.

Men may marry at age 18 and women at age 16 without the consent of their parents. A woman cannot remarry for 6 months following a divorce or death of her husband, presumably to determine the paternity of any possible pregnancy. This law has been under discussion for some time. The newly married couple may chose either the family name of the husband or wife, more commonly selecting the husband's. Marriages, births, property, and other vital data are then registered under the selected name. If the wife's family name is selected this is considered to be "adoption" of the son-in-law into the family line. With more working professional women wanting to keep their father's family name, the registration system has come into considerable question in recent years. Now some couples keep their "working names" that are recognized by their companies. However, without the official registration the wife and children do not have rights to the family line in any way. If there are children outside of marriage the child takes the mother's family name unless the father is willing to acknowledge the child.

In 1990, 5.9 persons per 1000 population were married. During the years 1970-74 there was a marriage boom. 10-10.5 per 1000 population were married at that time. Being single is presently fashionable for the younger generation. This is most likely due to an increase in the level of education for women. Women in their late 20s now select their own way of life. Marriage is not their final goal. In the past 5 years the unmarried rate has increased from 24% to 30%. Men who wish to marry are having difficulty finding a wife. Some men have difficulty becoming independent from their families, particularly their mothers. This may be a pathological phenomenon of a modern high technology society, it may be an extreme emotional bonded relationship, or it may be an expectation discrepancy of both the mother and the son.

Immediately following the war the average age of marriage was 26.1 years for men and 25.8 years for women. In 1989, the average age of marriage increased to 28.5 for men and 25.8 for women. Marriage in Japan is an expensive social custom. The cost of the wedding is shared by both families according to their ability to pay. Contribution of the wife's assets after the marriage is not clearly defined in law or in custom in Japan. Generally, prenuptial agreements are not made. In years past arranged marriages were most common and included many traditions, customs, and obligations. Presently, there is a tendency to introduce young people only when they become older than the average marriage age. In some cases families may make wedding arrangements without the agreement of the young couple. A woman may agree to a marriage, particularly if there is no brother to take the family name. In these cases the husband takes the name of the woman's family and is adopted into the family line.

Carrying on the family line is of particular significance in Japanese culture. Birth rate, total fertility rate, and age of mother are displayed in Table 16-12. Through the years the birth rate has decreased dramatically and first birth mothers have become slightly older. Intervals related to birth have remained relatively steady.

Short birth intervals and, more recently, mothers in the work place, have affected breastfeeding practices. Working mothers find breastfeeding difficult to continue. However, new legislation has been passed that supports mother's time off from work following childbirth. Data on breastfeeding prevalence and duration indicates an increase in both during the last 15 years (Table 16-13).

In 1990 the divorce rate in Japan was 1.28/1000 marriages. Most (90%) of the divorces are done by mutual consent. Only 10% contest divorces and go to court. In most cases the children live with the mother following a divorce. Children who carry on the family name have rights to property. Families managed by divorced persons constitute 3.6% of the population.

Divorced women and widows have more difficulty managing a home financially than households with husbands. Most women left alone are not skilled

Table 16-12. Birth Rate, Total Fertility, and Mean Age of Mother by Live Birth Order

| Year | Birth Rate/ 1000 | Total Fertility Rate | Mean Age of Mother | | | | Average Interval Between Marriage- 1st Birth | Average Intervals Between Births | |
			Total	1st Birth	2nd Birth	3rd Birth		1st- 2nd	2nd- 3rd
1950	28.1	3.65	28.7	24.4	26.7	29.4		2.3	2.7
1955	19.4	2.37	28.2	24.8	27.2	29.5	1.68	2.4	2.3
1960	17.2	2.00	27.6	25.4	27.8	29.9	1.79	2..4	2.1
1965	18.6	2.14	27.4	25.7	28.3	30.3	1.82	2.6	2.0
1970	18.8	2.13	27.5	25.6	28.3	30.6	1.81	2.7	2.3
1975	17.1	1.91	27.4	25.7	28.0	30.3	1.72	2.3	2.3
1980	13.6	1.75	28.1	26.4	28.7	30.6	1.79	2.3	1.9
1985	11.9	1.76	28.6	26.7	29.1	31.4	1.80	2.4	2.3
1989	10.2	1.57	28.9	27.0	29.4	31.7	1.86	2.4	2.3
1990	9.9	1.53							

Table 16-13. Breastfeeding Prevalence and Duration from 1975, 1980, and 1985

| Year and Feeding Pattern | Months of Feeding | | | | | | |
	0-1	1-2	2-3	3-4	4-5	5-6	6-7
1975							
Total		100.0	100.0	100.0	100.0		
Breastfeeding		45.5	39.8	33.7	27.3		
Artificial feeding		29.6	38.6	44.7	58.8		
Mixed feeding		24.9	21.6	21.6	15.9		
1980							
Total		100.0	100.0	100.0	100.0		
Breastfeeding		45.7	40.2	34.6	29.8		
Artificial feeding		19.3	30.4	40.5	52.2		
Mixed feeding		35.0	29.4	24.9	18.0		
1985							
Total	100.0	100.0	100.0	100.0	100.0	100.0	100.0
Breastfeeding	59.9	49.5	45.4	39.6	35.9	33.4	30.7
Artificial feeding	8.1	9.1	20.8	28.5	41.8	47.8	51.9
Mixed feeding	32.0	41.4	33.7	32.0	22.4	18.8	17.4

for jobs. Many must move from the family house due to difficulty making payments. Given high rental rates in Japan, women alone, particularly women with children, struggle financially. Many times children are financially unable to pursue higher education.

The government has responded to the special population with understanding and generosity. Beginning in 1969, fatherless families are eligible for special loans. Children of these families may also obtain special loans when they reach age 20.

Many cities provide counseling services within the ability to pay. Municipalities give preferential retail permits, including cigarette sales licenses, to members of fatherless families. Civil service jobs also give preferential treatment in hiring.

Welfare is available both in cases where the father has died and in cases where the mother needs assistance raising the children. In cases of death of the father the family is given about ¥5,000 (US $600) for the first child and an additional ¥16,000 (US $128) for each child per month. In cases of divorce there is a set amount. However, the social welfare law usually provides about ¥21,000 (US $168) for the first child and an additional ¥1,700 (US $14) for each child per month.

Besides these benefits. a special income tax deduction is available for widows and divorcees. Training courses are available for job preparation for divorcees. If the mother is ill and cannot go to work or care for the child, home care may be provided. If the case is extreme, the children can be placed in the home of a volunteer or kept in a child welfare facility until the mother is able to care for the child again.

WOMEN'S BEHAVIOR, SEXUALITY, AND CRIMES AGAINST WOMEN

Women's Behavior

The role of women in Japanese society is a fascinating paradox. On one hand women have an expected norm for public behavior that appears dependent and reserved, on the other hand women are powerful with regard to many social structures. Women's behavior is expected to be reserved and demure and, in the formal circumstances of an office or classroom, rather quiet. Behavior in Japan is mainly situational, not determined by a universally applicable set of standards. One learns how to behave in a great number of given situations. In general, women are not socially trained to be assertive or outspoken as are women in other countries. Particularly, women's language changes when talking to people who are more respected, equal, and younger rank. But there is no overall idea of behaving on principle or a general notion of how to behave in new and unusual circumstances.

Many professional women in Japan are as competent, assertive, and responsible as their female counterparts in other parts of the world. Women's organizations are a good example of the organizational and rational ability of women. In the household, also, women are in control. This includes family finances, education of the children, and household decision of many kinds. Most companies send the husband's monthly salary to the bank account which the wife controls or it is given directly to the wife. The wife gives her husband and children an allowance and is expected to manage the finances in an orderly competent way.

Sexuality

Women are primarily responsible for birth control both inside and outside of marriage. Condoms are the most common form of contraception in Japan and are available from pharmacies, grocery stores, and vending machines. Contraceptive cream is not commonly available, but contraceptive jelly is sold under the product name "FP jelly." Diaphragms, while not commonly used, are available without prescription at pharmacies. Diaphragm fitting and instruction is done by a gynecologist. IUDs are available at hospital outpatient departments and are inserted by a gynecologist. Injections are not available at this time.

Contraceptive pills can be obtained by prescription. They are primarily available for medical treatment such as menstrual irregularity. They are not commonly prescribed for contraception because the consensus of the medical community is that the side effects are too great. However, there is currently some pressure from pharmaceutical companies to make contraceptive pills more available. Table 16-14 indicates the contraceptive practices in 1988. Table 16-15 indicates the percentage of persons using common contraceptive measures.

Table 16-14. Contraceptive Practices in 1988.

Practice	Percent
Using contraception	56.3
Previously used contraception	19.6
Never used contraception	21.5
Others	3.6

Under the Eugenic Protection Law abortions are permitted by medical doctors for health and economic reasons until 24 weeks gestation. It is sometimes said that abortion is Japan's most common method of contraception. There has been a marked increase in teenage abortion. In the age group 12-15, 44.1% of fetal deaths were due to induced abortion. In the age group 16-19, 33.2% of fetal

Table 16-15. Percentage of Persons Using Specific Contraceptive Measures

Contraceptive Measure	Percent
Condom	76.8
Body temperature	9.7
Calendar	6.6
IUD	5.3
Coitus interruptus	4.9
Tubal ligation	5.8
Contraceptive pill	1.7
Vasectomy	1.6
Jelly	0.5
Diaphragm	0.0

deaths were due to induced abortion. Teenagers become aware of their pregnancies too late, fail to seek advice, or are not aware of the actual gestational age of the fetus. Recently the gestational age for abortion was changed from 24 to 22 weeks to address the problem of delayed teenaged abortion. Adult abortion rate is very high as well.

Crimes Against Women

As in many other countries, sex is an entertainment commodity and men are the usual buyers. Bath house brothels are often called soaplands. Pink salons are bars with hostesses that can often provide sex for money and are commonly located near large train stations displaying gaudy neon signs. Hostesses in bars and clubs are there to please male customers, most commonly by boosting frail egos with flattery and attention. Small stickers with provocative pictures, a phone number, price, and time length can often be found in phone booths.

Socialization with colleagues in the work place is an important part of the corporate culture. There is much pressure on employees in the work place to participate in evening activities that often include excessive drinking. These activities sometimes provide opportunities for sexual harassment. Women have difficulty avoiding these frequent company parties because they want to keep their jobs and cooperate with the socially expected behavior.

There are strict antipornography laws that include a Film Ethical Committee. The sexual pornography law in Japan prohibits showing pubic hair. Unfortunately, the letter of the law is strictly adhered to but the intent of the law is ignored. Many kinds of pornography are readily available with small patches over pubic hair or camera angles that avoid pictures of pubic hair. Pornographic videos are available at every neighborhood video rental store and hotel room. Many channels commonly show sexual activity on midnight television, often including violence against women. Magazines, cartoons, and daily newspapers commonly include not only nude photos but also photos of many sexual activities. Each includes the required patch covering pubic hair. There is a general air of indifference and lack of sensitivity to these insults to women. Many Japanese ignore this or feel that there is nothing wrong with this as long as the law is obeyed. Not surprisingly, many women accept this as norm.

Domestic abuse of women is quite common; however, there is a strong social taboo against recognizing and publicizing it. Recently, newspapers have begun to carry stories of wife abuse and incest. No clear data is available at this time either on wife abuse or incest. Rape cases are much the same. There were 1,556 reported cases of rape in all of Japan in 1989. When a wife files suit for divorce, abuse by the husband is the reason given in 36.4% of the cases, the second most common reason given. The first most common reason given in wife-initiated divorce is disharmony.

In 1989, there were 26,480 women in prison. This is 4.2% of all persons in prison. No data are available at this time on prison conditions for women or abuse of women in prison.

WOMEN'S POLITICAL AND SOCIAL STRENGTHS

Political Participation

In Japan, all citizens above age 20 are eligible to vote. There is no separate system of voter registration. Voting by women is only slightly lower than voting by men. However, data on voting age in the population show the numbers of women voters slightly greater than the numbers of men. Table 16-16 shows the percent of female and male voters in various types of elections.

Women participate in national and regional political parties and other organizations. Table 16-17 shows the number and percentage of women in the Diet at the national level. At least two of these are nurses and another nurse is presently preparing to run for office with the strong support of the Japan Nurses Association. Table 16-18 shows the number and percentage of women in regional political parties.

Although women are a minority in elected positions, they are gaining a strong influence on public policy. Deliberative councils are committees appointed by the national Diet to study and report back on controversial issues. The deliberative councils which include women have increased from 30.8% to 75.9% of all councils during five years. This is a remarkable increase of women on committees that have a strong influence on public policy.

Table 16-16. Percent of Males and Females Voting for Various Governmental Officials

Official	Female	Male
Prefectural governor	56.41	52.36
Prefectural assembly	62.40	58.45
Mayor of specified city	67.31	64.02
Assembly of specified city	54.56	48.98
Mayor	69.24	63.72
City assembly	68.13	62.45
Headman of specified ward	52.68	45.65
Ward assembly	52.46	45.40
Town headman	88.23	84.38
Town assembly	89.03	85.15

Table 16-17. Women in National Government in 1990

Statistic	Total	House of Representatives	House of Councilors
Total	762	510	252
Number of Women	46	12	34
Percentage	6.0	2.0	13.5

Table 16-18. Women in Regional Political Parties in 1990

Statistic	Total	Prefecture	City	Town, Village	Specified
Total	65,616	2,798	19,070	42,728	1,020
Number of Women	1,633	72	862	608	91
Percentage	2.5	2.6	4.5	1.4	8.9

During the 1991 unified election for regional public party members there were more women elected into the assembly than any other time in history. This success was largely due to participation of women in local politics supported by a network of women at the grassroots level. The issues that won them popularity were the urgent and concrete needs of the people. These needs included such problems as waste disposal, care of the aged, kindergartens, stimulating education, facilities for the handicapped, and others.

Women concerned about specific issues send delegations to lobby with political parties. Candidates recognize the value of women's votes and often aim their campaign platform to gain women's votes. One prefectural vice governor is a woman. There are two more women who are high officials in the government of Tokyo and in Okinawa.

In connection with the United National Decade for Women the number of women's politically active organizations and labor unions increased from 41 to 52. This includes 10 nongovernmental organizations that are politically active such as the Japan Nurse's Association and the YWCA. These organizations advocate special interests related to women.

In addition to women's political groups, there are a large number of volunteer women's social welfare organizations. Each has its own objectives but most raise support for philanthropic causes and give awards to public servants. Two of these are the Pilot Club, a group of professional women physicians, attorneys, and others, and the Foloptomist Club.

Women are presently serving in Japan's self defense forces. There is no draft into the self defense forces. Information about the roles women play in the military is not available at this time.

17

Women's Health Status in the Republic of Korea

WHO Collaborating Centre for Research and Training for Nursing Development in Primary Health Care Yonsei University College of Nursing

Hea Sook Kim

SYNOPSIS OF COUNTRY

The Korean peninsula is located at the eastern end of the Asian continent and extends southward among China, the Soviet Union, and Japan. Korea is roughly 1000 km (600 miles) long and 216 km (135 miles) wide at its narrowest point. This relatively small land is divided into the Republic of Korea in the south and the Democratic People's Republic of Korea, sometimes called North Korea, by the Demilitarized Zone at roughly the 38th parallel. The land area of the Republic of Korea is 99,200 square km (38,301 square miles) and its population is 43.5 million. Administratively, the Republic of Korea consists of nine provinces; one special city, Seoul; and the five metropolitan cities of Pusan, Taequ, Inch'on, Kwangju, and Taejon. There are 67 cities and 137 counties in the nine provinces.

The Koreans, whose ancestors used to live in northeastern Asia, mostly in Liaoshi, Manchuria, and the Korean peninsula, have developed into a highly homogeneous people. Ethnically, Koreans belong to the Mongolian race, but for centuries the people have maintained their unique language, culture, and customs.

The Korean language is regarded as a member of the Altaic family, which includes such languages as Manchurian and Mongolian. The Korean language, called Hangul, is comprised of 10 simple vowels and 14 consonants.

The Korean government is a centralized administration system which is governed by the president. Also, in 1991, a local governing system became operative.

In spite of Korea's commitment to a health insurance system for all Korean people by 1989, the rates of insurance coverage remain low. Furthermore, medical facilities and manpower are maldistributed between urban and rural areas. Thus the major health concerns of government are 1) prevention and management of chronic degenerative diseases and enhancement of health education, 2) stabilization of the health insurance system, and 3) optimization and equalization in the utilization of health services.

DEMOGRAPHICS

A woman's place in a society is a reflection of the culture of that society. In Korea, an understanding of the position of a woman must consider her role within the family or on her place within the community and the country as a whole. In the last three decades, Korea has experienced dramatic economic growth, accompanied by rising female labor force participation and substantial progress for women in living standards, health, and education.

The life expectancy for Koreans is 67.4 years for males and 75.4 years for females. By 1990, the crude birth rate had decreased from 29.9 in 1970 to 15.6 per 1000 people. The sex ratio was 101.3 men per 1000 women. Just over a quarter of the population (25.8 %) was under 15 years old, and 69.2% of the population was in the economically active years of 15-64. Although only 5.0% of the population today is over age 64, this age group is increasing rapidly as the nation's health improves.

As the death rate has declined, there has been a shift in the most common causes of death from respiratory and digestive illness to malignancy and cerebrovascular disease. The infant mortality rate decreased from 53 per 1000 live births in 1970 to 12.5 in 1988. The maternal death rate showed a similar downward trend, decreasing from 8.3 per 100,000 in 1970 to 2.9 in 1990.

HEALTH CARE SYSTEM

The health care system in Korea can be divided into two parts, the private sector and the public sector. For the majority of people, health care is provided by the private sector. People who are employed are covered by private health insurance, and as of July 1989 everyone in the country is covered under the national health insurance system.

The centralized administration for the public sector is the Ministry of Health and Social Affairs (MOHSA), which operates government hospitals at the city and provincial level and health centers at the country level. In Korea there are 249 health centers, focusing mainly on the delivery of preventive health services.

There are 588 hospitals in Korea, with a total of 98,501 beds. Of these, 35 are large private general hospitals of over 500 beds. Most of these hospitals are located in Seoul or other major cities; 83.3% of these hospitals are in cities. In the isolated rural areas where there are 70 medical facilities, 2,038 community health nurse practitioners (CHP) are working in health posts as part of the government's primary health care policy.

Health personnel include physicians, dentists, oriental medicine physicians, midwives, nurses, medical technicians, pharmacists, nurse's aides, and others. Nurses have a major role among the health professionals. In 1989, the number of certified nurses was 82,652, and 41,492 of them were employed as nurses. There is one nurse for every 513 people, based on all nurses certified. The number of physicians certified was 39,672, and 31,022 physicians were employed in 1989.

Indicators of Korea's social and economic development include a decrease in acute and infectious diseases owing to improvements in living conditions (e.g., implementing basic sanitary facilities). The Korean people are also assuming more responsibility for health management as evidenced by compliance with routine immunizations and medical treatments such as taking prescribed medication for acute and chronic illnesses. As the death rate and the birth rate have decreased and life expectancy has increased, elderly people over age 65 have increased in number. An increase in the elderly population has resulted in chronic degenerative disease as the main cause of death among the elderly.

HEALTH CARE UTILIZATION

The number of health programs in Korea has remained relatively low due to the emphasis on economic growth rather than social development since the 1960s. Despite the lack of attention to health issues, economic growth has resulted in the improvement of the women's health as well as of the general health of the public. Table 17-1 highlights specific aspects of women's health in Korea, including the rise in life expectancy for males and females, the increase in age at marriage and the decrease in childbearing, the increase in maternal child health services and the decrease in maternal and infant mortality, and the growing problem of single mother households and poverty.

Table 17-1. The Health Status of Korean Women

Category	1975	1980	1983	1986
General Health				
Life expectancy				
Female	66.7[a]	69.1		68.5
Male	59.8[a]	62.7		
Sexual composition rate (F/M)	101.2	101.8	102.1	
Morbidity rate				
Female	7.4	10.0	8.1	
Male	6.5	8.3	7.1	
Nutritional intake				
Calories	2390	2485	2588	
Protein (grams)	71.1	73.6	78.3	
Average age at menopause			47.6	
Later Marriage and Smaller Families				
Average age at first marriage				
Female	23.3	23.6	24.1	
Male	27.1	27.4	27.3	
Family planning rate of eligible women	44.2	54.5	70.3[b]	
Artificial abortion rate	39	49	50	
Ideal number of children	2.8	2.7[c]	2.5[d]	
Total birth rate	3.2	2.8	2.4	
Total stillborn rate	2.3	2.9	1.8	
Health in Childbearing				
Maternal mortality rate (per 100,000)	5.6	4.2	3.8	3.2
Infant mortality rate (per 100,000)	41.4	36.8	34.2	22.0
Prenatal care rate	57.2[e]	75.9	87.9	
Medically assisted delivery (%)		59.5	46.7	79.7
Economic Issues				
Number of female-headed houses		707,091	741,710	
Protection needed female-headed houses				
Number		65,946	73,857	
Percent		9.6	10.0	

[a]1970.   [b]1984.   [c]1978.   [d]1982.   [e]1977.

Sources: EPB, Social Indicators of Korea, 1983; The Ministry of Health and Social Affairs, Health and Social White Paper, 1984; The Population and Health Institute, Yearly Statistics on Population and Family Planning.

Today women's health issues and the involvement of women in health care are increasingly recognized as important for the society as a whole. Women not only have special health problems related to pregnancy and childbirth, but they also customarily have a major responsibility to care for family members and their health. Women's health has improved markedly in recent decades due to economic growth, an improved public conception of hygiene, better nutrition, and expanded medical facilities. The National Health Insurance Program, which expanded its coverage for all from July 1, 1989, has contributed significantly to the improvement.

In modern society, with increased participation of women in the labor force, the issue of maternity protection is emerging as a significant concern of the government, employers and trade unions. The Maternal-and-Child Health (MCH) Law, the Industrial Health Law, the Labor Standards Law, and the Child Protection Law were all enacted to safeguard mothers and infants. Article No. 44 of the Labor Standards Law defines six types of jobs forbidden to women for health reasons. Unfortunately, these laws have had less impact on maternal-child health than the lawmakers intended, at least partly due to the lack of public awareness of the concept of "maternal care."

Current measures designed to enhance the health of mother-and-child include the following:

a)   Offer registration and management services for expectant mothers and their fetuses.
b)   Offer delivery aid and supply expectant mothers with proper nutrition.
c)   Establish and operate MCH centers.
d)   Train MCH workers, and actively engage in such education and publicity.
e)   Launch the maternal physical protection program for working mothers on a continuous basis.

The government and health care system also support family planning programs designed to deter the population growth. Several strategies designed to achieve this goal include:

a)   Diversify the target group for family planning programs in both persons and areas.
b)   Upgrade and spread the use of contraceptives more widely.
c)   Provide differentiated application of medical insurance rates and social welfare programs in favor of the families which have fewer children.
d)   Reinforce research, evaluation, education, and publicity to deal with population policies.

Women's Health and Childbearing in Korea

Traditional Customs. Pregnancy is considered as a blessing because it continues the family blood line into the next generation. Therefore, an infertile woman is treated as an unqualified wife. The husband of a woman who is infertile is advised to have a baby through adoption from one of his brother's children or through a surrogate relationship. Sons are especially important because when one doesn't have a son, one cannot expect devotion after death through the ancestors' ceremony. Only a son can conduct the ceremony. Once a woman is pregnant, she is treated differently. She is exempted from participation in funerals, wedding ceremonies, and group meetings because she is considered unclean. A pregnant woman must take care of herself and do what is especially good for her baby. This is what we call *Taegyo* [fetal education]. *Taegyo* is a holistic approach to prenatal care. It was said that the mothers of famous, respectable ancestors did *Taegyo* diligently all through their pregnancies.

Health Care During Pregnancy. Child-bearing age women (15-49) formed 46.7% of the total female population in 1970 and 54.5% in 1985. More than 90% of married women experience conception and delivery, reflecting the high value placed on having children that continues today. The dramatic decline in both maternal and infant mortality (Table 17-1) reflects changes in the health care services provided to mothers and infants. Clinical delivery increased from 32% in 1977 to 85.8% in 1986, while home delivery dropped from 64.2% in 1977 to 12.9% in 1986. The rate of prenatal care has increased from 75.9% in 1980 to 93.8% in 1986, and the average number of prenatal visits has increased from 3.9 in 1980 to 5.9 in 1986.

Under the Maternal-Child Health Act, enacted in 1973 and revised in 1986, local administrative offices issue a medical check-up pocketbook to pregnant or nursing mothers. This guarantees medical examinations on a regular basis, pre- and postnatal care, and safe delivery. Newborn babies also receive free vaccinations.

Prenatal service is not covered by medical insurance in the hospital, health care center, or midwifery clinic. The cost of prenatal care in the health care center and midwifery clinic is comparatively lower than in the hospital. About 20.0% of women deliver their babies at home. These are mostly in the rural areas and they have access to some prenatal care from the community health practitioners, who are nurses practicing in the remote rural areas. The scope of prenatal service at the national health care center is very limited. But hospital physicians are providing diagnostic tests and examinations to ensure women have access to necessary prenatal care. Research is also being conducted to gather data necessary to improve prenatal health care.

Family Planning Methods. Since 1962 when family planning was started in Korea, we have focused on family planning methods for married couples in order to control the fertility rate and promote health care. Between 1970 and 1987, the national fertility rate dropped from 4.2 to 1.99 (Table 17-2). The greatest decline has occurred in the childbearing rate during the early twenties, but the rate has

Table 17-2. Changes in Age-Specific Marital Fertility Rate, Induced Abortion Rate, and Contraceptive Practice Rate, 1978-1987

Year and Item	All Ages	Age Groups				
		21-24	25-29	30-34	35-39	40-44
1978[a]						
Marital fertility rate (per 1000)	4.1	374	271	127	30	15
Induced abortion rate (per 1000)	2.9	70	156	148	156	54
Contraceptive use (%)	49	16	38	62	66	47
(Sterilization)	(16.5)	(1.8)	(11.9)	(24.4)	(24.9)	(12)
1985[a]						
Marital fertility rate (per 1000)	3.4	414	209	45	9	2
Induced abortion rate (per 1000)	2.1	92	149	115	40	20
Contraceptive use (%)	70	36	61	84	87	70
(Sterilization)	(40.5)	(8)	(29)	(52)	(58)	(43)
1987[b]						
Marital fertility rate (per 1000)	2.6	271	192	41	6	4
Induced abortion rate (per 1000)	1.6	102	103	71	29	7
Contraceptive use (%)	77	44	65	87	90	82
(Sterilization)	(48.2)	(9)	(30.5)	(59)	(65)	(59)
Percent Change 1987-1987						
Marital fertility rate (per 1000)	-36.6	-27.5	-29.2	-67.7	-80.0	-73.3
Induced abortion rate (per 1000)	-44.8	-45.7	-34.0	-52.0	-81.4	-87.0
Contraceptive use (%)	57.1	175.0	71.0	40.3	36.4	74.5
(Sterilization)	(192.1)	(400.0)	(156.3)	(141.8)	(161.0)	(391.7)

[a]Jong-Kwan Lim, "A Review on Induced Abortion in Korea," Journal of Population and Health Studies, 8(2), KIPH, 1988.

[b]KIPH, 1988 Fertility and Family Health Survey, Seoul, 1989.

declined for women at all ages. The proportion of married couples using family planning has increased by 23.4% over the past 10 years. The use of induced abortion has declined, while the use of sterilization has dramatically increased between 1978 and 1987.

Research has shown that increased information and communication between husband and wife have been influential factors for bringing about attitudinal changes among married couples, including an increase in the practice of family planning. Oh (1988) reported that the younger women and women who marry later have more husband-wife communication on family planning.

In the past, most husbands thought that family planning was the wife's responsibility. However, since 1981 this belief has begun to change. One of the reasons for the change has been the national residential policy, payment, and benefits. The government began to give priority in house allocation to families in which the father had been sterilized or who had a small number of children. A couple expecting their second child is given a free delivery once the husband has been sterilized.

EDUCATIONAL ACHIEVEMENT FOR WOMEN

Historically, Korean women's education was confined to the home. Only men were given any formal education, while women had the duties of looking after the home and bearing children to maintain the family line. *Instructions for Housewives*, written by Queen Sohye of the Yi Dynasty (1392-1910) and the first education for women in the country, outlines a code of conduct for housewives based on Confucian norms of a traditional society, calling on women to become affectionate mothers and good-natured wives. However, the emergence of the Sirhak (practical learning) in the middle of the 17th century and the Tonghak (Eastern learning) in the late 19th century influenced an expansion of the ideology of human rights and equality, regardless of social class or gender. This ideological base led to gradual changes in traditional norms and women's role. Meanwhile, missionaries introduced Western civilization into Korea around the 1880s.

Formal education for women began with the Ewha Haktang, Korea's first school for women, which was inaugurated in 1886 with the enrollment of only one girl student. Confucian culture and a national policy of isolation that dominated Korean society at that time made it difficult to establish and operate girls' schools. However, Christian missionaries managed to set up a number of middle schools such as Chongsin and Paewha Girls' Schools in Seoul and Sungin Girls' School in Pyongyang.

It was after the political reform of 1884 that Korea established public schools under a new educational system. The 1884 reform move recognized the need for education of women, but the school decree that was proclaimed had provisions for male schools only. The Adoration Society, founded in September 1898, with the objective of establishing and operating a girls' school financed by membership fees, announced in the same month "A Letter on Girls' School Facilities." This document was considered the country's first declaration of the rights of women with respect to education in that it was aimed at not only establishing girls' schools but also at attaining equal rights for both sexes.

The Republic of Korea Constitution prescribes that "All citizens shall have the right to receive equal education in accordance with their capabilities." Thus, one of the basic rights of citizens is to be accorded educational opportunities irrespective of sex, age, or class.

In 1985 men had an average of 9.66 years of education, while women had an average of only 7.58 years. A 6-year primary school course has been compulsory since 1949 when the Education Law was adopted. More than 90% of all children eligible for schooling, boys and girls, were enrolled in primary schools as early as the 1960s.

The ratio of primary school graduates advancing to middle school was 99.5% for girls and 99.6% for boys in 1988. The ratio of middle school graduates advancing to high school in the same year stood at 92.1% for girls and 94.9% for boys, showing little difference by sex. The ratio of high school graduates entering college and universities in 1988 was 32.7% for females and 37% for males. Of total enrollments in college and university in 1988, women accounted for 26.9%. Almost as many girls as boys attend primary and secondary school, but the proportion of women decreases substantially in college and graduate school. The percentage of female students by educational level in 1991 is presented in Table 17-3.

Table 17-3. Percentage of Female Students by Education Level, 1991

Education	Total	Number of Females	Percent of Females
Nursery/Kindergarten	414,532	196,842	47.5%
Elementary School	4,868,520	2,362,050	48.5%
Middle School	2,300,978	1,106,516	48.1%
High School	2,346,736	1,110,383	47.3%
College/University	1,403,898	433,951	30.9%
Graduate School	86,911	19,560	22.5%
Total	11,421,575	5,229,302	45.8%

Source: Statistical Yearbook of Education 1990.

In an effort to meet the increased demand for skilled manpower, vocational high schools provide education and training in more than 90 courses. In 1988, girls accounted for 51.2% of the enrollment in vocational high schools, but in technical high schools the proportion of girls was only 1.4%, while in commercial schools it was 77.8%. Among students taking 4-year college courses, subjects preferred by women are different from those chosen by male students. Majors preferred by female students in 1988 were, in the order of preference, arts, teaching, language and literature, medical and pharmacy, sciences, and social sciences. Arts accounted for 64.3% and teaching for 55.3%. Preferences among male college students were engineering, followed by social sciences, medical sciences, language and literature, and teaching. These figures show there still are traditional prejudices against female students who choose more technical courses, science, and mathematics.

The Ministry of Education directed the 5th School Curriculum Study council to review sexual prejudices in curricula. Accordingly, contents of textbooks being used in schools from 1989 were revised on principles of equality between sexes. Technical crafts for male students and home economics for female students were merged into one subject. Since 1987 it has been offered to both boys and girls in middle and high schools. Along with the revision of curricula, efforts are being made to change teachers' sex discriminatory teaching attitude.

To cope with the rapid changes taking places in an industrialized society and recognizing the limits of school education, life-long education has been promoted in recent years. Non-formal education was institutionalized under the Non-Formal Education Law promulgated in December 1982. Under the law all citizens are accorded life-long opportunities for education.

ECONOMICS

In the past 15 years, there has been remarkable improvement in the standard of living of Koreans and in their health standards. The per capita GNP grew from $304 in 1970 to $4,994 in 1989. During this same period, the admission rate to universities increased from 7.6% of the high school graduates to 43.8% in 1988.

Increased Labor Force Participation

The participation of women in social activities today is at a higher level than ever before, especially in economic fields. It is a well-known fact that the remarkable economic growth Korea has achieved in the past two decades owes much to the female labor force in the manufacturing sector. Women are expected to make an even greater contribution to future economic development in view of the changing structure of industry and employment.

The size of the female labor force fluctuates in relation to population, participation in economic activities, and wages. In terms of the supply to the labor force, the female population gradually decreased from the 1960s and now stands in the neighborhood of 1.57%, and is expected to drop further to around 1.2% in the year 2000. However, the ratio of female participation in economic activities increased. Among the country's female population 15 years old and over, the proportion who were economically active increased sharply from 26.8% in 1960 to 45.7% in 1975, then fell to 38.4% in 1980, and has since started to increase, up to 45% in 1988. The decline in women's participation in economic activities in the latter half of the 1970s was attributed to the economic recession in the wake of the oil crisis.

Women's economic participation is greater in rural areas than in urban areas (52.9% versus 38.8%). Labor force participation rates are especially high for rural women age 30 and above. This indicates that the rural areas suffered a shortage in the labor force as males and young girls migrated to the cities and industrial areas, and the gap created was filled in large part by middle aged housewives. This reflects a feminization of farming labor during a period of rapid industrialization and urbanization.

In cities, the participation of married women in economic activities has shown a gradual increase. A number of factors are believed to account for this increase. First, women are receiving more years of education than in the past, so they are not starting to work at such early ages. Hence, the gap is being filled by middle-aged women. Second, an increase in living standards and educational expenses for children has prompted housewives to earn money to supplement their husbands' incomes. Third, women have a stronger desire to take part in social activities and can adapt to careers more readily than their predecessors.

In addition to the quantitative increase in women's economic activities, there has been a structural change in female employment. The proportion of women workers engaged in primary industry has declined in recent years in contrast with increases in the secondary and the tertiary sectors. In 1988, about 22.9% of women workers were still engaged in the primary sector of agriculture and fishing. About 29.2% of women workers were in the secondary sector (manufacturing) and 47.9% were in the tertiary or service sector.

About 80% of female workers in the manufacturing sector are employed by textile, clothing, electric, and electronic industries, which have led the nation's exports since the 1970s. Most of them are young and unmarried, so that women aged 14 to 44 account for 53.9% of the female labor force in the manufacturing industries.

Over the past two decades increasing numbers of women are taking clerical jobs. Women in clerical occupations accounted for 11.3% of the whole female work force in 1988, in comparison with 1.1% in 1965. These jobs continue to be dominated by young, unmarried women workers. The proportion of female employees in professional, technological, and administrative jobs increased from 1.5% in 1960 to 6.2% in 1988. This indicates that the level of education acquired by women has been upgraded due to the increased educational opportunities. But the rate of increase needs to be accelerated in order to respond to the increasing number of women graduates from schools of higher education.

Discrimination and Women's Work

Over the last several decades, the level of education acquired by women who work has been increasing. As indicated in the Table 17-4, women with higher

Table 17-4. Employed Women's Educational Attainment and Occupation, 1987

		Educational Attainment			
Occupation	Total	Under Middle School	High School	Junior College	College and University
Professional and Technical	5.0	0.4	4.3	56.1	70.5
Administrative and Managerial	0.0	0.0	0.1	0.0	0.5
Clerical	10.0	0.8	35.8	22.7	15.5
Sales	17.0	16.5	21.0	8.3	6.7
Service	14.2	14.7	14.7	6.1	4.2
Agriculture, Forestry, and Fishingman	35.2	47.5	6.1	2.3	0.5
Manufacturing and Related workers	18.6	20.1	18.0	4.5	2.1
Total	100.0%	100.0%	100.0%	100.0%	100.0%
Number	5,610,000	3,983,000	1,340,000	132,000	93,000

Source: Economic Planning Board.

levels of education are generally in higher level occupations. Those with less than a high school education work mainly in farming and manufacturing, while high school graduates are mainly in clerical, sales, and other service occupations. The majority of women with at least junior college educations are in professional occupations. However, only a small proportion of women in Korea have been able to enter managerial and high level administrative jobs, even among college and university graduates.

However, social and cultural conditions still are unfavorable for women with higher education in regard to participation in economic activities. As the number of women with college education has increased, the proportion of them who are employed has decreased, from 50% in 1980 to 37% in 1990. Equally important, among those college graduates who are employed, the proportion working in professional level jobs has decreased from 79% in 1980 to only 47% in 1990. One quarter of the female college graduates working in 1990 are working at clerical level jobs (Table 17-5). There has been a small but important increase in the proportion in managerial jobs, from 1.2% to 4.5% in 1990.

Table 17-5. Changing Trends in Economic Activities of Women Employees Among College Graduates (Percent)

Group	1980	1985	1986	1987	1988	1989	1990
Graduates	100.0	100.0	100.0	100.0	100.0	100.0	100.0
Higher degree course	8.9	6.1	4.8	4.7	5.1	6.1	6.1
Employed	50.3	29.8	26.8	27.4	29.7	33.9	37.3
Unemployed	23.5	42.0	46.4	46.0	44.1	43.9	41.6
Other	17.3	22.2	22.1	21.9	21.1	16.1	15.0
Occupation	100.0	100.0	100.0	100.0	100.0	100.0	100.0
Professional	79.0	48.1	52.7	46.7	45.8	47.6	47.2
Administrative	1.2	2.8	5.2	5.3	4.8	5.1	4.5
Clerical	11.3	17.2	19.8	22.1	23.4	23.4	25.0
Sales	4.6	12.0	9.3	11.4	12.1	12.2	11.8
Agriculture, Forestry	0.2	0.5	0.6	0.9	0.4	0.8	0.6
Production	2.1	1.3	1.6	1.4	0.9	1.1	0.9
Other	1.7	7.9	7.2	12.0	12.6	9.7	10.5

Source: Mnistry of Education, Statistical Yearbook of Education (1991).

It is clear that most of the increase in female employment came in simple and unskilled work, and increases in female employment in professional and skilled jobs and in administrative and supervisory positions are smaller than that of the male sex. As more women receive higher education and as they are better motivated to engage in economic activities, it is anticipated that an increased number of educated and experienced women will engage in professional and skilled work and take administrative and supervisory posts.

Official statistics indicate that women workers are still facing sexual discrimination in the labor market such as restrictive recruitment practices, lower wages, and limited opportunities for promotion. In an effort to alleviate such discrimination, the Equal Employment Opportunity Act was established in 1987, and was enforced in April 1, 1988. The act guarantees basic equality between men and women in employment, and special provisions for pregnancy and maternity with one-year child care leave as well as 60 days paid maternity leave.

The act also imposes the duty upon employers to provide child care facilities in work places.

The occupational structure for Korean women by age shows a pattern closely related to child care. Working women with infants are burdened with the dual responsibilities of a job and a home. To maintain female employment without interruption and to ease the burden on married women employees, it is necessary to expand nursery facilities at the job site as well as in the community. With this in mind, the government incorporated a plan for women's development in the Sixth Five-Year Economic and Social Development Plan launched in 1987. Envisaged under the plan were the establishment of nursery facilities at job sites and the introduction of a child care leave system under which female employees could leave to rear their infants and then later return to their jobs. Studies are also in progress to examine the benefits of employing women on a part-time basis. If such social and institutional support were provided, women would be able to offer a more specialized and stable labor force in a wide range of fields, as well as make a contribution to society.

FAMILY STRUCTURE

Household Type

The total number of households in Korea has been increasing since 1966. In 1985 the number of households reached 9,571,361, an increase of 3,204,361 or 30.3% over 1975. In terms of household type in 1985, two-generation households accounted for 67.0%, three-generation households 14.4%, one-generation households 9.6%, and one-person households 6.9% (Table 17-6).

Trends of Marriage and Divorce

The average marriage age has increased in portion to the number of years women spend in school. Women's average age at the time of their first marriage increased from 21.6 in 1960 to 25.3 in 1988 while men's average age increased from 25.4 in 1960 to 28.4 in 1988. In 1988 there were 409,000 marriages recorded, and the marriage rate was 9.85 per 1,000 persons. The number of divorces in 1988 was 44,000 and the divorce rate was 1.05 per 1,000.

Monthly Income

Employment conditions for women are still considerably inferior to those for men. In 1971 the average monthly payment of female workers was 277,610 won, which was 54.1% of that of male workers. The average monthly payment of female workers increased 23-fold during the last two decades, but the gradient in

Table 17-6. Changes in Household Type per 1000 Households, 1966-1985

Type of Household	1966 N (%)	1970 N (%)	1975 N (%)	1980 N (%)	1985 N (%)
One generation	278 (5.5)	376 (6.7)	447 (7.0)	659 (8.3)	916 (9.6)
Two generations	3,316 (65.6)	3,906 (70.3)	4,580 (71.9)	5,547 (68.5)	6,412 (67.0)
Three generations	1,179 (23.3)	1,230 (22.1)	1,278 (20.1)	1,312 (16.5)	1,383 (14.4)
More than three generations	127 (2.5)	64 (1.1)	62 (1.0)	42 (0.5)	60 (0.4)
One person	117 (2.3)			383 (4.8)	661 (6.9)
Unrelated persons	34 (0.7)			117 (1.5)	160 (1.6)
Total	5,052 (100.0)	5,576 (100.0)	6,367 (100.0)	7,969 (100.0)	9,597 (100.0)

Source: EPB, Population and Housing Census Report, 1966, 1970, 1975, 1980, 1985.

the income levels of males and females has not been significantly lessened. The gap between levels of income among males and females continues to reflect discrimination against women.

Women and Law

The Constitution of the Republic of Korea, which was proclaimed in 1948, includes regulations for the equality of men and women and the prohibition of sexual discrimination. Article 10 declares that "All citizens shall be equal before the law and there shall be no discrimination in political, economic, civic, or cultural life on account of sex, religion, or social status." Article 36(1) states "Marriage and family life shall be entered into and sustained on the basis of individual dignity and equality of the sexes." It guarantees all citizens, both men and women, the right to vote or be elected to public office under conditions prescribed by law. It also stipulates that all citizens shall enjoy freedom of occupation and have the right to work. Special protection is accorded to working women, and unjust discrimination in terms of employment, wages, and working conditions is prohibited. In spite of those constitutional provisions, certain laws sanction unequal treatment of men and women.

The revision of the Family Law in December 1989 was the most significant breakthrough to date in improving the legal status of Korean women. The Law had been controversial for the past 30 years and contained discriminatory provisions rooted in old traditions. Women's organizations had made concerted efforts to revise the law, and as a result the law was revised in 1977, and again in 1989.

Although not all the proposed revisions were made in the law, it currently provides for the equal status of women in the family, especially in the area of property. The following is a summary of the revised provisions:

- The designation of head of the family remains, but the provisions on the succession of the family head status are deleted.
- Child custody upon divorce is no longer automatically granted to the father. Rather this right is determined either by the couple's mutual agreement or by the Family Court.
- The domicile is to be decided by both parents and not by the husband only. The wife and the husband have equal responsibility for living expenses.
- Women's rights of inheriting property are also expanded. The revised law eliminates discrimination against daughters. When there is no will, the properties can be distributed evenly among the children regardless of sex. A childless widow is now entitled to get half of her husband's inheritance, with the remaining half going to his parents.
- Both wife and husband have equal rights to the properties gained after marriage and have the right to ask for an equal division of properties. The law thereby entitles a divorcing woman to seek a share of the couple's property in proportion to her contribution to its accumulation.
- The relatives are defined as within third cousin for both mothers and fathers.

Although the revision of the Family Law contributes a great deal to promoting the legal status of women, it still contains provisions on the leadership of the family and the prohibition of marriage between persons of the same origin and surname.

WOMEN'S STRENGTHS

Women and politics

Under the Constitution of the Republic of Korea promulgated in 1948 and which declared equal rights for both sexes, women have enjoyed equal rights with men before the law. Women have been given the right to vote, to run for election, to assume public duties, and to affiliate with political parties.

Exercising equal rights with men, women have so far participated in 13 general elections to choose legislators, 13 presidential elections, and 6 national referenda. Of eligible women voters, 80.6% used their franchise in the presidential elections, while 85.1% of eligible men voted. In the general elections, 72.9% of eligible women and 76.6% of eligible men voted. The women's vote increased from 70.5% in the 1963 general elections to 76.3% in the 1981 general elections, reflecting an increase in political awareness among women.

Since the inauguration of the Republic of Korea in 1948, a total of eight women have been appointed as cabinet members. Of a total of 726,089 civil servants in 1988, 23.2% were women, of whom 58.5% were teachers in public schools.

The higher the job rank, the smaller the number of women. Only 0.5% of civil officials of rank 5 and above were women in 1988. The proportion of women among political party members shows a sharp increase in recent years as does the actual number of women party members.

In the ruling Democratic Liberal Party the ratio of men to women is 6 to 4. The opposition Peace and Democracy Party has a woman vice president. Efforts are being made to increase the number of women members on influential decision-making party organs, including educational programs designed to upgrade the leadership and political consciousness of women party members.

Women's group activities, once largely geared toward leisure and friendship promotion, especially among the middle class, expanded their functions to include substantial interests concerning women's advancement in Korean society. Newly established women-related organizations with specific agendas and organizational strength set the courses of the women's movement as a larger social movement by working to increase women power in society. Existing women's organizations are changing in terms of "Content and Formality" and have reinvigorated group activities through in-depth analysis of organizational, financial, and management strategies.

Another change during the 1980s was the growth of women's consciousness through various cultural means. Women pursued alternative cultural avenues such as literature, drama, movies, and art to address problems stemming from a male-dominated culture.

Women's advancement is also evident in such communications areas as newspapers, broadcasting, books, and other publications. As of the end of March 1990, however, women involved in such mass communications as daily newspapers, broadcasting, and other news agencies numbered only 3,530, or 11.3% of the total. Most female producers and reporters are assigned to departments concerning life, culture, and art, and kept away from political, economic, and social reporting. Problems involving promotion and sexual discrimination continue to exist. Still worse, the image of women represented by mass media sticks to the traditional notion of separate sex roles, and femininity tends to be commercially abused. Thus, the immediate need is to bring about sexual equality and a healthy culture through women's self-determination.

Women and Women's Research Institutes in Korea

The following list presents research topics and associated research institutes committed to the study of women's issues in Korea:
A. Joint Research on Women
    Korean Association of Women's Studies
B. Research on Establishment of Korean Women's History
    Korean Women's Institute of Ewha Women's University
C. Welfare Policies for Alienated Women
    Research Center For Asian Women of Sookmyung Women's University
D. Research on the Employment of Female University Graduates
    Women's Study Institute of Seoul Women's University
E. Symposium and Research on Sex Roles
    Women's Studies Center of Busan National University
F. Development of a New Curriculum on Women's Studies
    Women's Studies Center of Busan Women's University
G. Research on Household Labor
    Women's Problems Research Institute of Hyosung Women's University
H. Concentrated Research on Family and Women
    Women's Society for Korean Social Research
I. Women's Studies by Sessions of Labor and Literature
    Korean Society of Women's Studies

Government Employment by Sex and Organization

Women are usually in special posts such as counseling and health care which have limited opportunities for promotion. Out of a total of 801,870 civil servants in 1991, 24.2% were women, of whom 59.8% were teachers in public schools.

Women's Organizations

Women's participation in interest groups is also a good indicator of the political status of women. Women's non-governmental organizations (NGOs) can exercise influence on political decision-making and mobilize public opinion on women's issues. Registered women's organizations to the Government numbered more than 70 in 1990. It is believed that the number surpasses 100 with the inclusion of unregistered organizations.

Women's organizations are engaged in a wide range of activities in accordance with the objectives of their establishment. Included among them are the education of adult women to develop their abilities and make constructive use of their leisure time; social campaigns aimed at reinforcing the consciousness of women and improving their social standing; counseling designed to resolve women's problems arising from family conflicts; revision of The Family Law, which contains sex-discriminating provisions; and consumer protection drives, which tackle problems that arise through the process of industrialization and economic development.

While some organizations have been successful, most organizations suffer from financial difficulties and organizational problems. As of 1990 there were 17 organizations that received financial assistance from the Government. In the future, women's organizations need to overcome problems in organization, finance, and problems. They must make concerted efforts to reinforce their role as pressure groups, press for increased participation by women in the decision-making process of national policies, and become active agents of social change.

POLITICAL PARTICIPATION OF WOMEN

Ministry of Political Affairs

The Ministry of Political Affairs is in charge of women's affairs, particularly those related to women's participation in various social, economic, and political activities.

Administrative System for Women's Affairs

In addition to the Ministry of Political Affairs, there exist individual bureaus and divisions established under other ministries to deal with women's affairs so that women's rights may be properly protected in the process of policy implementation by each ministry.

Korean Women's Development Institute

The Korean Women's Development Institute was established in April 1983 as a national research center to study women's affairs. It is fully funded by the government and undertakes comprehensive research projects related to women. Among other activities, it provides education and training programs to enhance women's skills and abilities and initiates various action-oriented programs concerning women.

Women's Development Plan

Korea ratified the UN Convention on the Elimination of All Forms of Discrimination against Women in December 1984. Following the ratification, the government inaugurated the Women's Development Plan as a separate section along with 30 other sections in the Sixth Five-year Socio-Economic Development Plan (1987-1991).

LEGISLATION AND POLICIES TO IMPROVE THE STATUS OF WOMEN

Family Law

The revision of the Family Law in December 1989 was the most significant breakthrough to date in improving the legal status of Korean women. The Law had been controversial for the past 30 years, and women's organizations had made concerted efforts to revise the law, which was regarded as the most serious example of institutionalized discrimination against women.

The revised law provides for the equal status of women in the family, especially in the area of property. In relation to the revision of the law, the Inheritance Tax Law, which was adopted by the legislature in 1990, increased the standard for the inheritance tax deduction accorded to the spouse, based on the recognition that an unemployed spouse, especially a housewife, also has significant property rights.

Child Care Act

The new Child Care Act was legislated and put into effect in August 1991. Child care centers supported by the government for low-income families are now being operated at 250 different locations throughout the country. Through the Apartment Rental Program for female workers, started in 1981, the government has provided a total of 1,775 apartment units to accommodate 8,875 women as of January 1991.

Education and Training

Career Guidance for Girls. As a long-term strategy to eliminate sexual discrimination, it is important to provide education at an early age to change traditional attitudes toward women. The government operates special programs for female high school students to promote positive attitudes towards a career. The career guidance programs are classified into separate programs for teachers and parents and for female students. In 1990, the government developed a Model Career Guidance Program for middle school girl students and disseminated it to the Education Committees of cities and countries. In the future, the government plans to develop guidelines for students at other levels of education.

The government also sponsors a program entitled "The World of Professions" on the newly established Public Education Broadcasting Station to encourage girl students to acquire a healthy and enlightened attitude toward careers.

Women's Studies Course for Civil Servants and Teachers. The government now includes a new course on Women's Studies in the training of civil servants and teachers at the national and public training institutes. The purpose of the new policy is to eliminate sexual prejudices held by civil servants and teachers who exercise significant influence in Korean society so that their attitudes on sexual equality can spread to other parts of society.

Social and Political Participation. The government is committed to providing women with opportunities and information concerning volunteer activities. The government is in the process of developing volunteer programs for housewives with light childcare responsibilities and proper experience and expertise. At the present time there are 180 women's volunteer activity centers in the nation which provide a linkage between the volunteers and the public agencies that are in need of volunteers.

The Ministry of Political Affairs provides active support to women's organizations that are concerned with social issues. The Association of the Women's Movement for a Better Society, which was formed voluntarily in June 1990 by more than 70 women's organizations, has carried out campaigns to help solve the problems that have a direct impact on the social development of Korea. So far, the Association has carried out a street campaign to save energy in 272 areas. Approximately 43,000 women have participated in this effort. Other activities of the Association have been a movement to combat drugs and pornography, a movement to protect the environment and to save clean water, a campaign for helping the less fortunate, and a campaign to restore morality.

The proportion of female participants in the policy-making committees of the government has increased from 2.2% in 1984 to 9.0% in 1990. It is the goal of the government to increase the figure to 15% by the year 2,000. The Ministry of

Political Affairs provides a list of women candidates to relevant government agencies, aiming at the goal of 10% female participation in 1991.

Health: Pre- and Post-Natal Maternity Leave. To promote women's health, the government has made all pregnant women eligible for the benefits of maternity health care programs of public health centers. In 1991, the government issued "The Standard Guidelines for Practicing Pre and Post-Natal Maternity Leave" for the purpose of strengthening the maternity protection of working women.

Social Welfare, Health, and Social Activities. The Apartment Rental Program for Single Female Workers, which began in 1981 as a social welfare program, has been successful in providing a total of 7,025 apartment units to accommodate 35,125 women in the 1980s. In addition, from 1990 to 1992, 1,000 apartment units will be built every year to benefit a total of 10,025 women.

By the end of 1990, there were a total of 1,919 daycare centers in the nation accommodating 48,000 children. This number falls far short of the demands for daycare centers. In order to meet this need and to provide systematic daycare, the Child Care Act was legislated in January 1991. The law provides a legal basis to establish government-sponsored daycare centers for low-income working parents and private daycare centers for other children. It is expected that 2,010 government-sponsored daycare centers for low-income children and 32,210 private daycare centers for children will be established by 1995.

Women's health has improved substantially in recent decades due to economic growth, improved public awareness of hygiene, better nutrition, and expanded medical facilities. For example, the ratio of the child deliveries carried out at hospitals increased to 88.9% in 1988 from 68.8% in 1983. The maternal death rate decreased from 5.0 per 1,000 births in 1976 to 3.9 in 1988. The infant mortality rate stood at only 12.1 per 10,000 in 1987. The Welfare Act for Fatherless Families legislated in April 1989 will contribute to the further improvement of women's health.

In the process of modernization and democratization, women's participation in social activities has become quite active, both quantitatively and qualitatively. Today there are more than 2,000 women's organizations in Korea. Considering the fact that there were merely 23 organizations in the 1960s, the quantitative growth in the 1980s is truly impressive. The scope of activities ranges from purely social and cultural interests to campaigning against sexual discrimination in law and in practice. The Ministry of Political Affairs maintains close relations with these groups to survey public opinion and to formulate its own policies, and also to provide them with financial support.

The Ministry of Political Affairs has promoted active cooperation with international organizations and individual women leaders abroad. As Korea becomes a new member state of the United Nations, it will do its best to contribute to the system of international peace and cooperation developed through the United Nations. Korea has participated in the various meetings of the Commission of the Status of Women held in Geneva as an observer and expressed its concerns regarding women's development. After the ratification of the Convention to Eliminate All Forms of Discrimination Against Women, Korea submitted to the United Nations two reports on the status of women in Korea.

STATUS OF KOREAN WOMEN

In the traditional society of Korea, women's role was confined to the home. Women were required to follow the Confucian virtues of subordination and endurance, and they were denied opportunities to participate in political and social activities. Their major function was to give birth to offspring to preserve the family line, and women served to maintain the order of the family under the extended family system. In terms of both social status and hierarchy, women were inferior to men. Regardless of social status, social institutions and the custom of avoiding the opposite sex did not permit women to be involved in non-family affairs.

The situation began to change, however, thanks to the educational opportunity for women that followed the opening of the country to the outside world in the 1880s. Educated women engaged in arts, teaching, and religious work, as well as enlightening other women on the problems of poverty and illiteracy. The self-awakening of women led to their national awakening under Japanese colonial rule, and women took part in the independence movement with no less vigor and determination than men. A liberation movement calling for human rights for women also began to emerge.

With the promulgation in 1948 of the Republic of Korea Constitution guaranteeing equal rights for both sexes, women began to obtain equality under law. After gaining the right to vote, to be elected, and to assume public duties, women were able to participate in the country's major policy making processes. Although their political rights came in recognition of the stand and actions of women in the struggle for the country's independence and enlightenment, it could be said that suffrage for Korean women came relatively easily compared to their Western counterparts who acquired the franchise only after long struggle.

With the successful implementation of the Fifth Five-Year Development Plans since the early 1960s, Korea has achieved remarkable economic growth. Export-oriented industries required a large female labor force. As the society diversified and the educational level of women was raised, demands for skilled and professional women increased. Despite the increase in the number of women engaged in social and economic activities, it has not been easy to resolve women's problems arising from traditional values and institutions. Some inequalities persist in access to non-traditional education and occupations, equality of pay, poverty of single mothers, inadequate child care services, and the stress of continued traditional home obligations as well as work in the formal sector. Korean women will continue to work for improvement in their overall status in society, and this will promote continued improvements in women's health.

REFERENCES

Han, Jung-Ja (1985). Women's organizations' activities in Korea, *UN Evaluation of Women in the Decade.* Korean Women's Associations United.

Korean Legal Center. (1984). *Laws of the Republic of Korea* (4th ed.).

Korean Overseas Information Service. (1990). *A handbook of Korea,* 478-491.

Korean Women's Development Institute. A study on laws related to women's welfare. *Research Report 200-3,* 79-137.

Korean Women's Development Institute. (1985, July). *Status of women in the Republic of Korea.* Paper presented to the world conference of the UN for women.

Korean Women's Development Institute. (1991). The present situation of Korean women's organizations. *Women's Studies Forum, 7,* 245-283.

Korean Women's Development Institute. (1991). *Reference on Women,* 400-15.

Korean Women's Development Institute (1991). A study for trends of men-women employee's ratio in productive areas. *Research Report 200-4.*

Korean Women's Development Institute Newsletter. (1989). Women of Korea—Present status and future prospects. Office of the Minister of State for Political Affairs, Republic of Korea, 1-17.

Korean Women's Development Institute Newsletter. (1991). Korean women today. No. 30, 1-3.

Korean Women's Development Institute Newsletter. (1991). Korean women today. No. 31, 1-7.

Korean Women's Development Institute Newsletter. (1991). Korean women today. No. 32, 1-7.

Kwon, Young ja. (1987). Networking for the development of women. *Journal of Asian Women 26,* Center for Asian Women of Sookmyong Women's University.

Ministry of Health and Social Affairs, Republic of Korea. (1990). *Yearbook of health and social statistics,* No. 35.

Ministry of Health and Social Affairs, Republic of Korea. (1991). *Yearbook of health and social statistics,* No. 36.

Conclusion

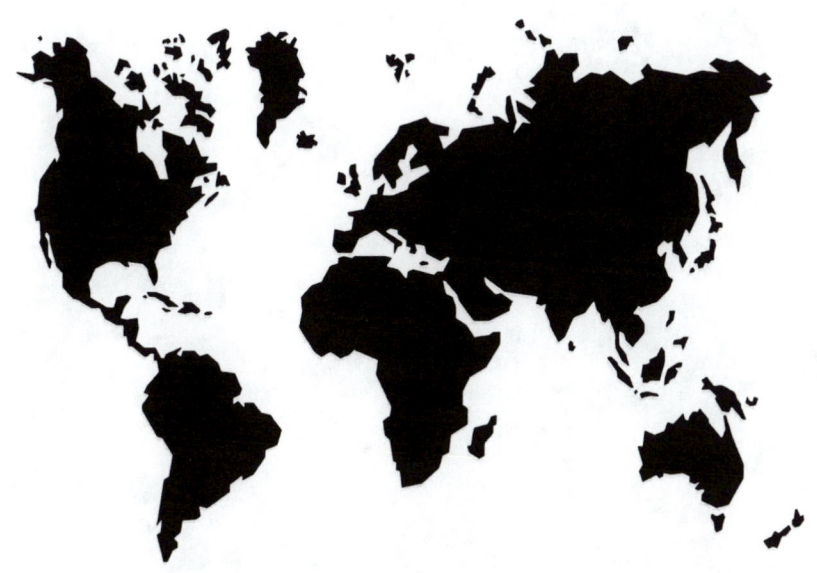

Investing
in the
Future

18

Women's Health Status: Investing in the Future

Miriam J. Hirschfeld

Assembled here are reports from the World Health Organization's Global Network of Collaborating Centres concerned with the development of nursing and midwifery. There are now some 27 such Collaborating Centres, distributed in 6 geographical regions.

The World Health Organization designates Collaborating Centres to support and enhance its work aimed at supporting national health development through the improvement of information resources, services, research, and training. A major part of this effort contributes to promoting women's health, the status of which is the subject of this document.

In a recent progress report on WHO regional and global activities in support of action by Member States to promote women's health and enhance the role and participation of women in development (WHO/FHE/WHD/92.5), the Director-General of WHO, Dr. Hiroshi Nakajima, emphasizes that women's health is fundamental to the development of a country.

To report points out some key actions to meet the challenge of improved health for women:

- expanding, improving and restructuring present primary health care and general health care and family planning services for all in order to make them financially more efficient, particularly in the light of the prevailing economic situation;

- providing specific health services for women's specific needs, complementing the existing ones and making them geographically and psychosocially accessible and acceptable, and ensuring the full participation of women themselves;
- providing women, their families and the public at large with information about women's health needs, problems and solutions;
- training health workers at all levels to take into account the perspectives of women and to provide health care and other appropriate means for the "carers," the majority of whom are women; and
- promoting and implementing research and data collection on behavioral, sociocultural, and economic aspects affecting the health of women, and operational research in cost-effective alternative interventions for both global priority health needs and problems of women such as reproductive health, including safe motherhood, family planning, prevention of sexually transmitted diseases, nutrition, reproductive cancers, and mental and occupational health.

As we look to the future, I am confident that the nursing Collaborating Centres will pursue an integrated research, education, and practice agenda that ensures the advancement of women's health as an important investment in human health and development. We must also look towards developing useful means for monitoring the progress in women's health at global, national, and grassroots levels. As the Director-General's report recommends, we can achieve better health for women through strengthening alliances between governmental and nongovernmental organizations and examining the allocation of resources and priorities that guide our work.

It is imperative that women become fully and effectively integrated into the development process, for to conclude with a final excerpt from the Director-General's report:

In the 1990s approaches to women's concerns will need to shift from the sidelines of development to a concerted initiative to bring women into the mainstream, to promote the role of women as agents of change; to make their health and social needs a top priority; and to equip them with equal access to information, technical and economic resources, skills, education, and opportunities, not only to benefit women in their own right, but to benefit all people and future generations.

REFERENCES

World Health Organization. (1992). *Women Health and Development: Progress Report by the Director-General.* Geneva, World Health Organization (WHO/FHE/WHD/92.5).

Appendix

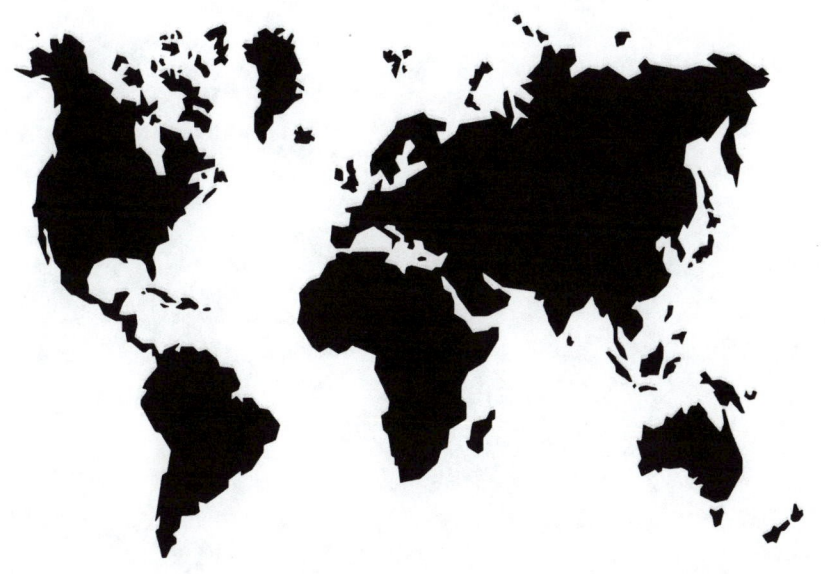

The Fifth International Congress on Women's Health Issues: Copenhagen, Denmark August 28, 1992

CONGRESS STATEMENT

This Fifth International Congress on Women's Health Issues recognizes the interactive relationship between health and the environment. 350 participants from 31 countries agreed that health is first and foremost determined by adequate economic and social conditions which assure sufficient food, water, shelter and other resources necessary for sustaining life and promoting health. Health is determined by the interaction of economic, political and social forces. Understanding the significance of this interaction means an appreciation of the interconnectedness between models of development being pursued in the world and systems of domination which reduce the capacities of people, especially poor people, to sustainably lead their lives.

The following recommendations follow from these facts:

Health work should be based on the recognition that human health cannot be protected and improved without protecting the eco-systems that sustain all life.

Social, political, and economic justice at global and national levels needs to be fundamental to health policy.

Democratization and decentralization of knowledge, resources, and decision-making are essential for attaining health for all.

Education for empowerment and occupational opportunities is fundamental for improving health.

Unnecessary and harmful medicalization of health practices needs to be exposed and stopped.

Human beings all over the world should work against dumping of harmful and useless drugs, tobacco products, reproductive technologies and industrial and toxic waste by the industrialized countries in the less technologically developed countries.

In the present, increasing unipolar world, UN organizations like UNEP, WHO, UNICEF, FAO, UNIFEM, and the Commission for Refugees need to be strengthened, reformed and sensitized to women's health issues worldwide. This includes greater representation of women at all organizational levels, including top leadership positions.